# Step by Step®
# ULTRASOUND IN GYNECOLOGY

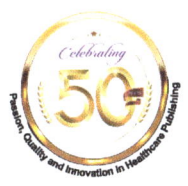

# Step by Step®
# ULTRASOUND IN GYNECOLOGY

**Third Edition**

### Editor-in-Chief
### Narendra Malhotra
MD FICMCH FICOG FRCOG FICS FMAS FIAP
President, INSARG, Past President, FOGSI/IFUMB/ISPAT/ISAR
Vice President, WAPM/SAFOG
Managing Director, Global Rainbow Health Care and MNMH (P) Ltd
Agra, Uttar Pradesh, India
Professor, Sarajevo School of Science and Technology, Croatia

### Associate Editors
### Nidhi Gupta
MS FICMCH FICOG
Past President, Agra Obstetrical and Gynecological Society
Professor, Department of Obstetrics and Gynecology
Sarojini Naidu (SN) Medical College, Agra, Uttar Pradesh, India

### Neharika Malhotra
MD (Gold Medalist) DRM (Germany) FICMCH Fellow ICOG (Rep Med) ICOG (USG)
Joint Secretary, FOGSI, Chair, YTP Committee, FOGSI
Director and Consultant, Global Rainbow IVF and MNMH (P) Ltd
Agra, Uttar Pradesh, India

### Jaideep Malhotra
MD FICMCH FICOG FRCOG FRCPI FMAS
President, SAFOM/ISPAT, Past President, IMS/ISAR/FOGSI/ASPIRE
Managing Director, ART—Global Rainbow IVF and MNMH (P) Ltd
Agra, Uttar Pradesh, India

### Kuldeep Singh
MBBS FAUI FICMCH
Consultant Ultrasonologist
Dr Kuldeep's Ultrasound and Color Doppler Clinic, New Delhi, India

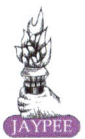

## JAYPEE BROTHERS MEDICAL PUBLISHERS
*The Health Sciences Publisher*
New Delhi | London

# Jaypee Brothers Medical Publishers (P) Ltd

**Headquarters**
Jaypee Brothers Medical Publishers (P) Ltd
EMCA House, 23/23-B
Ansari Road, Daryaganj
New Delhi 110 002, India
Landline: +91-11-23272143, +91-11-23272703
+91-11-23282021, +91-11-23245672
Email: jaypee@jaypeebrothers.com

**Corporate Office**
Jaypee Brothers Medical Publishers (P) Ltd
4838/24, Ansari Road, Daryaganj
New Delhi 110 002, India
Phone: +91-11-43574357
Fax: +91-11-43574314
Email: jaypee@jaypeebrothers.com

**Overseas Office**
J.P. Medical Ltd
83 Victoria Street, London
SW1H 0HW (UK)
Phone: +44 20 3170 8910
Fax: +44 (0)20 3008 6180
Email: info@jpmedpub.com

Website: www.jaypeebrothers.com
Website: www.jaypeedigital.com

© 2021, Jaypee Brothers Medical Publishers

The views and opinions expressed in this book are solely those of the original contributor(s)/author(s) and do not necessarily represent those of editor(s) of the book.

All rights reserved. No part of this publication may be reproduced, stored or transmitted in any form or by any means, electronic, mechanical, photocopying, recording or otherwise, without the prior permission in writing of the publishers.

All brand names and product names used in this book are trade names, service marks, trademarks or registered trademarks of their respective owners. The publisher is not associated with any product or vendor mentioned in this book.

Medical knowledge and practice change constantly. This book is designed to provide accurate, authoritative information about the subject matter in question. However, readers are advised to check the most current information available on procedures included and check information from the manufacturer of each product to be administered, to verify the recommended dose, formula, method and duration of administration, adverse effects and contraindications. It is the responsibility of the practitioner to take all appropriate safety precautions. Neither the publisher nor the author(s)/editor(s) assume any liability for any injury and/or damage to persons or property arising from or related to use of material in this book.

This book is sold on the understanding that the publisher is not engaged in providing professional medical services. If such advice or services are required, the services of a competent medical professional should be sought.

Every effort has been made where necessary to contact holders of copyright to obtain permission to reproduce copyright material. If any have been inadvertently overlooked, the publisher will be pleased to make the necessary arrangements at the first opportunity. The **CD/DVD-ROM** (if any) provided in the sealed envelope with this book is complimentary and free of cost. **Not meant for sale**.

**Inquiries for bulk sales may be solicited at:** jaypee@jaypeebrothers.com

*Step by Step® Ultrasound in Gynecology*

*First Edition*: 2004
*Second Edition*: 2010
*Third Edition*: **2021**
ISBN: 978-93-89587-42-5

*<u>Dedicated to</u>*

All the ultrasound lovers

# Preface to the Third Edition

*"Use sound to see better*
*Turn on the color to improve your image*
*Shift to the 3rd and 4th dimensions*
*Heal with sound"*

Ultrasound has evolved to a new generation from the Ian Donald's 1D to 4D. Today, diagnosis of the female pelvic disorders are not possible without a transvaginal scan (TVS).

The TV scan is quick, economical, reliable, reproducible modality for complete pelvic diagnosis. Addition of color and 3D and 4D on the transvaginal probe has provided more physiological and structural information.

After the overwhelming response of the first and second edition, we have come out with the third edition.

We have added few chapters like ectopic pregnancy, trophoblastic disease in first trimester, Intrauterine contraceptive device (IUCD), vaginal bleeding with negative pregnancy test and chronic pelvic pain as these problems make up a great volume for which the patients visit the gynecologists.

More than 60 algorithms and treatment flowcharts for common problems encountered by gynecologists have been added as a ready reckoner for the busy practitioners.

This edition aims to simplify the transvaginal scanning procedures and use it for better patient diagnosis, care and treatment.

**Narendra Malhotra**
**Nidhi Gupta**
**Neharika Malhotra**
**Jaideep Malhotra**
**Kuldeep Singh**

# Preface to the First Edition

Ultrasound today is the most accepted investigation and diagnostic modality for evaluating disease of virtually any and all parts of our body. Newer developments in technology have led to development of endocavity probes and high resolution clear pictures.

The advantages for Gynecological pelvic evaluation by transvaginal ultrasound are many folds and obvious. A high frequency probe placed near the target organ to be scanned gives us a clear anatomic picture of the uterus, cervix, ovaries and adnexa. Addition of color gives us physiological information about vascular supply. 3D and 4D give us sculpture like realistic images.

TVS is the only quick, cheap, reliable and reproducible modality to evaluate Gynecological problems.

**Kuldeep Singh**
**Narendra Malhotra**

# Acknowledgments

Our heartiest thanks to our parents, elders, teachers, spouses, siblings, our sons, daughters and our friends who have helped us step by step at every step of our ambitious project of step by step series.

We were introduced to interventional sonography by Ananda Kumar (Singapore), Rajat Goswamy (UK), Asim Kurjak and Sanja Kupesic (Croatia), Professor Alfred Kratrochwil (Austria), Ashok Khurana, Ambarish Dalal, Pratap Kumar, Bhupendra Ahuja, Dr PK Shah, Jatin P Shah and Pranay Shah and many others who taught us small tricks of the trade at each step of our life.

We are indebted to Professor Struat Campbell and Professor Asim Kurjak for teaching us imaging and grateful to Ian Donald School, India and INSUOG.

Special thanks to Dr Rahul Gupta and Nitin Agarwal of Rainbow 4D imaging center for all the images.

Editor-in-Chief
**Narendra Malhotra**

# Contents

1. Basics in Ultrasonography 1
2. Training 51
3. Introduction 55
4. Normal Anatomy of Female Pelvis 59
5. Pelvic Sonography 62
6. Normal Female Pelvis 69
7. Uterine Disorders 95
8. Ovarian Disorders 154
9. Miscellaneous Disorders 179
10. Ectopic Pregnancy 195
11. Trophoblastic Disease in First-trimester 210
12. Intrauterine Contraceptive Device 215
13. Vaginal Bleeding with Negative Pregnancy Test 221
14. Chronic Pelvic Pain 230
15. Common Gynecological Diseases 241

*Index* 301

# CHAPTER 1

# Basics in Ultrasonography

## BASIC PHYSICS

In order to obtain the best image possible, basic fundamentals of ultrasound wave physics must be understood and applied.

## Audible Sound Waves

Audible sound waves lie between 20 and 20,000 Hz: Ultrasound uses sound waves between l and 30 MHz.

## Sound Wave Propagation

Sound waves need a media to travel and do not exist in a vacuum, and propagation in gases is poor because the molecules are widely separated.

The closer the molecules are, the faster the sound wave moves through a medium, so bone and metals conduct sound exceedingly well.

### Effect on Image

Air-filled lungs and gut containing air conduct sound so poorly that they cannot be imaged with ultrasound instruments. Structures behind them cannot be seen.

A neighboring soft-tissue or fluid-filled organ must be used as a window through which to image a structure that is obscured by air.

An acoustic gel must fill the space between the transducer and the patient, otherwise sound will not be transmitted across the air-filled gap.

Bone conducts sound at a much faster speed than soft tissue.

Because ultrasound instruments cannot accommodate the difference in speed between soft tissue and bone, current systems do not image bone or structures covered by bone.

## Pulse-Echo Principle (Figs. 1.1A and B)

Because the crystal in the transducer is electrically pulsed, it changes shape and vibrates, thus producing sound waves that propagates through the tissues.

The crystal emits sound for a brief moment and then waits for the returning echo reflected from the structures in the plane of the sound beam.

When the echo is received the crystal again vibrates, generating an electrical voltage comparable to the strength of the returning echo.

### *Effect on Image*

Greyscale imaging shows echoes in varying levels of grayness, depending on the strength of the interface.

## Beam Angle to Interface (Fig. 1.2)

The strength of the returning echo is related to the angle at which the beam strikes the acoustic interface. The more

## Basics in Ultrasonography

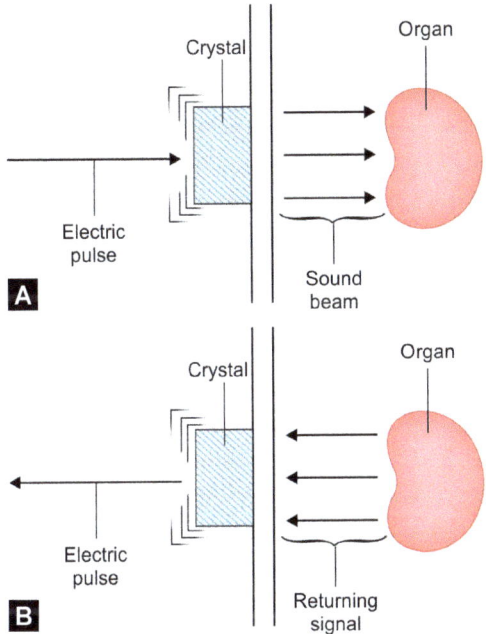

**Figs. 1.1A and B:** The pulse-echo principle. (A) The electrical pulse strikes the crystal and produces a sound beam, which propagates through the tissues; (B) Echoes arising from structures are reflected back to the crystal, which in turn vibrates, generating an electrical impulse comparable to the strength of the returning echo.

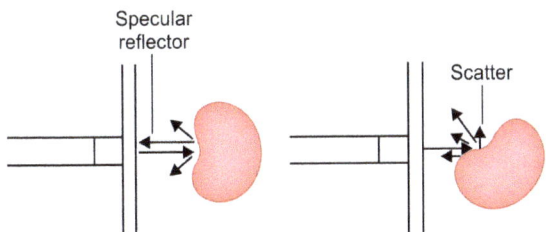

**Fig 1.2:** Beam angle to interface.

nearly perpendicular the beam is, the stronger the returning echo will be smooth. Interfaces at right angles to the beam are known as *specular reflectors.*

Echoes reflected at other angles are known as *scatter.*

### *Effect on Image*

To demonstrate the borders of a body structure, the transducer must be placed so that the beam strikes the borders more or less at a right angle.

It is worthwhile to attempt to image a structure from different angles to produce the best representation. **(Fig. 1.3)**.

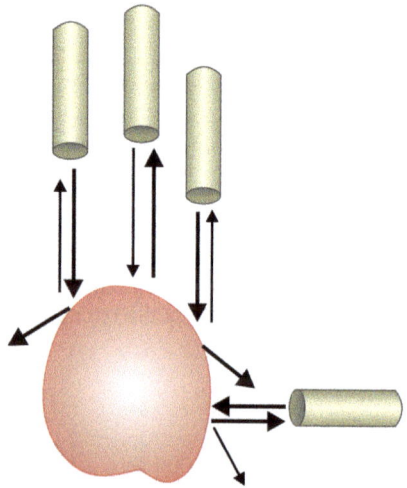

**Fig. 1.3:** When visualizing a structure, it is important to scan at several different angles to find the best possible interface *(thick arrows).* Only a few echoes return from the interfaces at an oblique angle to the beam—specular reflections *(thin arrows).* Most of the echoes are scattered.

# Basics in Ultrasonography

## Tissue Acoustic Impedance

The returning echo's strength also depends on the differences in acoustic impedance between the various tissues in the body.

Acoustic impedance relates to tissue density; the greater the difference in density between two structures, the stronger the returning interface echoes defining the boundaries between those two structures on the ultrasound image will be.

### *Effect on Image*

Structures of differing acoustic impedance (such as the gallbladder and the liver) are much easier to distinguish from one another than are structures of similar acoustic texture (e.g. kidney and liver).

## Absorption and Scatter

Because much of the sound beam is absorbed or scattered as it travels through the body, it undergoes progressive weakening (attenuation).

### *Effect on Image*

Increased absorption and scatter prevent one from seeing the distal portions of a structure. In obese patients, the diaphragm is often not visible beyond the partially fat filled liver.

Fibroids may absorb so much sound that their posterior borders may be difficult to define.

## Transducer Frequency

Transducers come in many different frequencies-typically 2.5, 3.5, 5, 7, and 10 MHz.

Increasing the frequency improves resolution but decreases penetration.

Decreasing the frequency increases penetration but diminishes resolution.

### *Effect on Image*

Transducers are chosen according to the structure being examined and the size of the patient. The highest possible frequency should be used because it will result in superior resolution. Pediatric patients can be examined at 5–10 MHz.

Lower frequencies (e.g. 2.5 MHz) permit greater penetration and may be needed to scan larger patients.

## Beam Profile (Fig. 1.4)

The sound beam varies in shape and resolution.

Close to the skin, it suffers from the effect of turbulence, and resolution here is poor. Beyond the focal zone, the beam widens.

### *Effect on Image*

Information that appears to be present in the near field may actually be an artifact. Structures beyond the focal zone are distorted and difficult to see. A structure as small as a pinhead may appear to be half a centimeter wide.

## Transducer Focal Zone

Sound beams can be focused in a similar fashion to light. Most systems use electronic focusing which permits the transducer to be focused at one or more variable depths. The sonographer can alter the focus level electronically.

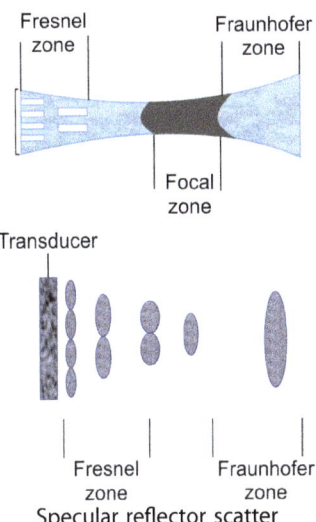

**Fig. 1.4:** Diagram of the waveforms in a sound beam. Unequal waveforms in the near field (Fresnel zone). Widening of focal beam (Fraunhofer zone) beyond the focal zone.

### *Effect on Image*

To achieve high resolution chose a transducer with a proper focal zone or use a electronically focusing set at the right depth.

## INSTRUMENTATION

## Transducers

The transducer assembly consists of five main components **(Fig. 1.5).**
1. The *transducer crystal* is composed of a piezoelectric material, most commonly lead zirconate titanate. It

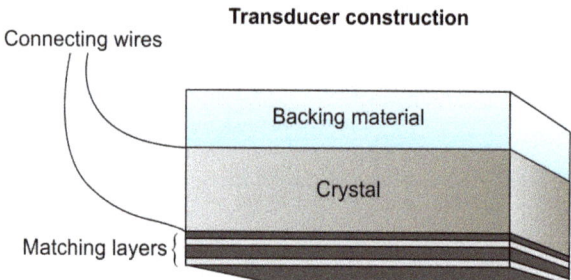

**Fig. 1.5:** Diagram showing transducer construction. Matching layers of material decrease the size of the main bang acoustic interface that occurs between the crystal and the skin. Backing material acts as a damping tool to stop secondary reverberations of the crystal. The crystal is constructed of piezoelectric material, which can convert electrical impulses into sound waves and vice versa.

converts the electrical voltage into acoustic energy upon transmission and acoustic energy to electrical energy upon reception.

2. The *matching layers* lie in front of the transducer element and provide an acoustic connection between the transducer element and the skin.
3. *Damping material* is attached to the back of the transducer element to decrease secondary reverberations of the crystal with returning signals.
4. The *transducer case* provides a housing for the crystal and damping layer and insulation from interference by electrical noise.
5. The *electronic cable* contains the bundle of electrical wires used to excite the transducer elements and receive the returned electrical impulses.

There are several types of transducer elements:

Basics in Ultrasonography

1. Mechanical transducers
   - The transducer crystal is physically moved to provide steering for the beam
   - Less commonly used in modern equipment than phased-array transducers
   - Often used in volume transducers for 3D or 4D applications.
2. Oscillating transducer (volume)
   - The drive motor and transducer array are housed in the transducer case
   - The motor drives the transducer array back and forth to generate an image **(Fig. 1.6)**.
3. Electronically steered systems
   - In this type of transducer, multiple piezoelectric elements are used and a separate electrical signal is provided for each element

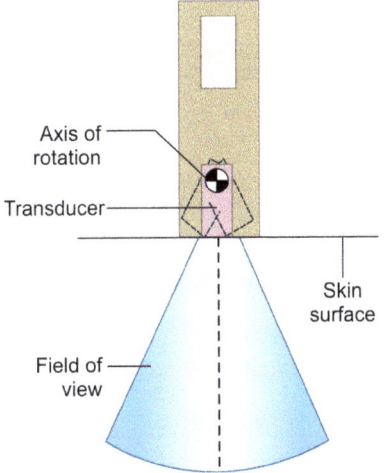

**Fig. 1.6:** Oscillating transducer (volume).

- Steering and focusing occur by sequentially exciting individual elements across the face of the transducer
- Focusing is controlled electronically by the operator through placement of the focal zone or focus caret
- The images are displayed in a sector, vector, linear, or curved linear format.

a. Linear sequenced arrays **(Fig. 1.7)**
   - Multiple transducer elements are mounted on a straight or curved bar.
   - Groups of elements are electronically pulsed at once to act as a single larger element
   - Pulsing occurs sequentially down the length of the transducer face, moving the sound beam from end to end
   - Linear arrays produce a rectangular shaped image which is used in breast, small parts, vascular, and musculoskeletal imaging
   - Curved arrays provide a large fan-shaped image with a curved apex. These transducers are most commonly used in obstetric, gynecologic, abdominal, and endocavity imaging.

b. Phased array
   - The phased array consists of multiple transducer elements mounted compactly in a line

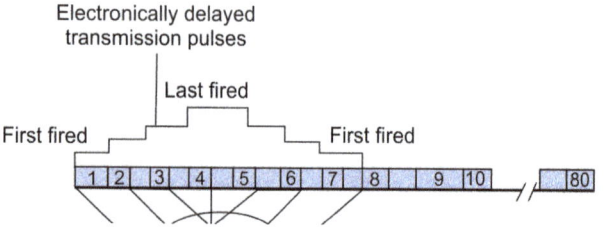

**Fig. 1.7:** Linear sequenced array.

# Basics in Ultrasonography

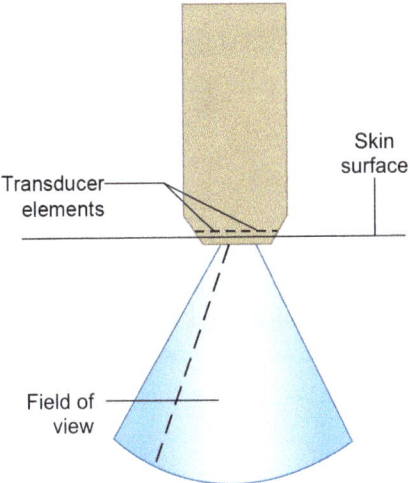

**Fig. 1.8:** Wedge-shaped field.

- All elements are pulsed as a group with small time delays to provide beam steering and focusing
- The resulting image is in a sector or vector format and is particularly useful in cardiac and intercostal imaging **(Fig. 1.8)**.

**Matrix Array (Multi-O Array, 1.5D Array, 2D Array) Transducers**:

- This type of transducer utilizes multiple rows of elements to form a matrix of crystals **(Fig. 1.9)**
- Through the use of multiple pulses, these crystals may be pulsed in sequence to create a very thin elevation plane (slice thickness), which yields increased resolution.

## Hanafy Lens Technology

- This is another technique used to create a very thin slice thickness that is uniform throughout the field of view

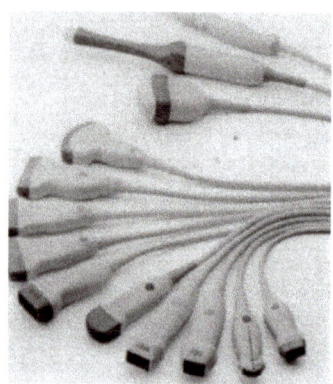

**Fig. 1.9:** Various ultrasound transducers.

- With this technology, the transducer crystals are cut in a planoconcave fashion **(Figs. 1.10A and B)**, which creates crystals that are thin in the center and thicker at the edges
- The thinner center will ring at a higher frequency (focusing in the near field), and the thicker edges will ring at a lower frequency (focusing in the far field), automatically creating a uniform elevation plane (slice thickness) throughout the field of view.

## Special Transducers

Special transducers **(Fig. 1.11)** have been produced to help view specific areas:
- Small parts (7.5-15MHz) transducer
- Rectal transducers in longitudinal (linear) and transverse (radial) configurations (biplane)
- Biopsy transducer
- Doppler probes.

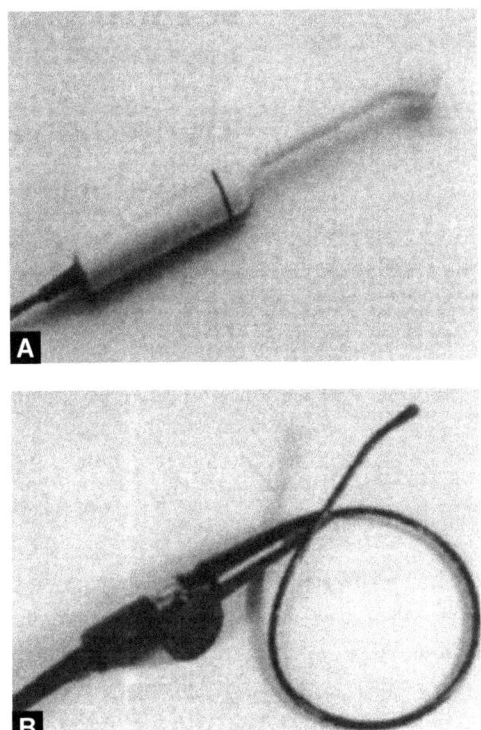

**Figs. 1.10A and B:** Transvaginal transducer. Transeophageal echocardiography transducer.

## Endocavity Ultrasound Systems

The transducer array, which can be a linear, curved, or phased array (or mechanical sector) scanner, is placed at the end of the transducer shaft. This transducer shaft is inserted into the rectum or vagina to produce high-resolution images of the male or female pelvic organs.

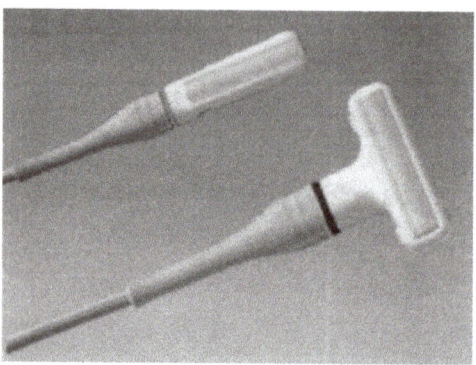

**Fig. 1.11:** Intraoperative transducers are designed to allow easy access to anatomy.

## Transesophageal Transducers

A transesophageal transducer may be introduced into the esophagus to visualize the heart and provides a higher resolution image than does transthoracic echocardiography.

## Intraluminal and Intracardiac Transducers

- Smaller transducers at the ends of catheters can be introduced into vessels, the biliary duct, or the ureter (transluminal transducers)
- These transducers allow close visualization of the anatomy that is being examined, but are not commonly used
- Intracardiac catheters have been developed more recently. A small catheter (IOF or *BF)*, which may be introduced into the right heart, provides very high-resolution imaging and may be used for interventional and electrophysiology applications.

## Operative Systems

Standard ultrasound systems are modified so they can be used in a sterile fashion in the operating room. Special high-frequency ultrasound probes are used for this purpose. Intraoperative transducers are designed with a size and shape to allow easy handling and positioning during intraoperative procedures.

## Transducer Formats

There are a variety of transducer formats available in modern equipment, each suited to particular scanning applications.

***Linear array:*** The linear format provides a rectangular image. This transducer is most useful in "small parts" and vascular imaging.

***Vector:*** A vector format provides a trapezoidal image. This small foot-print transducer is often used in abdominal, gynecologic, and obstetric applications.

***Sector:*** The sector image is wedge-shaped and is commonly used in cardiac, abdominal, gynecologic, obstetric, and transcranial imaging.

***Curved array:*** A curved array transducer will provide a large field of view with a convex near field. This transducer is most commonly used in obstetrics; however, other applications include abdominal and gynecologic imaging.

## NEW TECHNIQUES FOR IMPROVING THE IMAGE

## 3D Imaging Systems

- 3D imaging capabilities have been increasing in popularity' over recent years
- It is most commonly used in obstetric and cardiac imaging to evaluate the surface of structures or to evaluate orthogonal planes

- It utilizes specialized transducers which relate the transducers position to the ultrasound system allowing for a very accurate display of the acoustic echoes.

## 4D Imaging Systems

- 4D imaging systems use specialized transducers to display the real-time motion of a 3D image
- These are most commonly used for obstetric and cardiac applications
- The transducers are commonly mechanical transducers, which are held in place while the ultrasound system controls the acquisition of the images by "rocking" the transducer crystals and displaying the 4D images.

## Harmonic Imaging

- Images are obtained from returning signals, which are a multiple of the transmitted (fundamental) frequency
- The harmonic signal is created from the compression and relaxation of tissues during sound propagation
- It is helpful to reduce noise and clutter in an image, especially in technically difficult patients; however, harmonic imaging may suffer from decreased penetration due to the higher receive frequency.

## Tissue Harmonic Imaging and Pulse Inversion

- With traditional ultrasound techniques, the ultrasound system transmits a pulse of a specific frequency and receives a pulse of the same frequency. This frequency is known as the *fundamental frequency*
- As this fundamental frequency travels through tissues, the tissues compress and expand with the variations in

acoustic pressure, resulting in the generation of additional ultrasound frequencies, known as *harmonics*

- The harmonic frequencies are multiples of the transmitted fundamental frequency
- The challenge for the ultrasound system is to separate the clean harmonic signals from the fundamental signals. Tissue harmonic imaging removes noise from images, especially in patients who are difficult to image
- The simplest separation method is to lengthen the transmitted pulse
- Pulse inversion techniques utilize multiple pulses on transmit which vary in phase, which is maintained on transmit and receive
- The harmonic signals generated by the tissue have a different shape and phase than that of the transmitted pulse
- By summing the received pulses, the ultrasound system cancels the fundamental frequencies (destructive interference) and adds the harmonic signals (constructive interference)
- This technique often results in reduction in frame rate.

# Image Compounding

Multiple ultrasound frames are averaged together to produce an image with increased contrast resolution.

## *Compound Imaging/Sie Clear Multiview Spatial Compounding/Sona CT Cross Beam Imaging*

Image compounding averages multiple ultrasound frames to produce an image with increased contrast resolution.

Image compounding may use image frames of varying frequency (transmit or frequency compounding) or by utilizing image frames from varying angles (spatial compounding). They are of the following types:

### *Frequency Compounding*

Frequency compounding uses multiple transmit pulses to obtain images of the same area with different frequencies
- It provides an increase in contrast resolution and penetration.

### *Spatial Compounding*

- This technique interrogates the same area of interest from various locations
- By averaging these ultrasound frames, the speckle pattern is reduced and will provide an image with increased contrast resolution
- Spatial compounding may occur by varying the transmitted beam's location, varying the transducer position, or by varying the location of the receive beam.

### *Speckle Reduction Imaging*

Speckle reduction imaging is processing algorithm that reduces image speckle. The resultant images appear smoother and have increased contrast resolution as compared to the image without speckle reduction.

### *Elastography*

- Elastography is an ultrasound technique used to evaluate the relative stiffness of tissue as compared to the surrounding area
- Results may be qualitative or quantitative in nature.

**Compression elastography:** It is a qualitative imaging technique that utilizes manual compression to present the relative stiffness of tissue through a color or black/white overlay of the image. It is most commonly used in breast imaging.

***Shear-wave elastography:*** It is a technique that utilizes an electronic push pulse to provide compression of tissues. The speed of the shear wave generated by the tissue compression may then be measured. It is most commonly used in the evaluation of the liver.

## KNOBOLOGY

Learning to use the knobs effortlessly is an important part of the art of ultrasound imaging.

### Gain

The system gain controls the degree of echo amplification or brightness of the image. Care must be taken with the use of gain. Too much overall gain can fill fluid-filled structures with artifactual echoes, whereas too little gain can negate real echo information.

### Depth Gain Compensation

The depth gain compensation (DGC) attempts to compensate for acoustic loss of sound waves by absorption, scatter, and reflection and to show structures of the same acoustic strength with the same brightness, no matter what the depth is.

### Dynamic Range (Dynamic Contrast/Log Compression)

The dynamic range (log compression) is the range of intensities from the largest to the smallest echo that a system can display. Changing the log compression does not affect the number of gray shades in the image; instead, it varies the display of the gray shades.

## Edge Enhancement (Preprocessing)

The preprocessing control alters the edges of the image pixels to accentuate the transition between areas of different echogenicities, making the borders sharper.

## Frequency Selection (MultiHertz)

Frequency selection allows the user to optimize the imaging for the best resolution or penetration. Increasing the frequency will improve resolution but sacrifice penetration.

## Maps (Postprocessing)

Maps alter image esthetics by placing more or less emphasis on specific echo intensities. Changing the map may aid the user in evaluating pathology.

## Persistence

It is a frame-averaging function that allows echo information to be accumulated over a longer period of time. By increasing the persistence subtle tissue texture differences will be enhanced and by decreasing it the moving structures are evaluated more easily.

## Speckle Reduction Imaging

Speckle reduction imaging (SRI) is an image processing algorithm that reduces image speckle for enhanced contrast resolution. Higher SRI settings result in images with a smoother appearance and increased contrast resolution, as compared to the image without speckle reduction.

## Zoom

The zoom function allows image magnification by increasing the pixel size, although this change results in image degradation.

## Write Zoom (Res)

With write zoom, a box is placed on the screen, and the area seen within the box can be expanded to fill the screen.

## Transducer Selection

The transducer selection feature allows the user to activate the transducer of choice.

## Calipers

Caliper markers are available to measure distances. The ellipsoid measurement is an added feature in most units. A dotted line can be created around the outline of a structure to calculate either the circumference or the area.

# DOPPLER AND COLOR FLOW PRINCIPLES

Doppler physics as it relates to diagnostic ultrasonography concerns the behavior of high-frequency sound waves as they are reflected off moving fluid (usually blood) **(Fig. 1.12)**.

## Doppler Effect

When a high-frequency sound beam meets a moving structure, such as blood flow in a vessel, the reflected sound

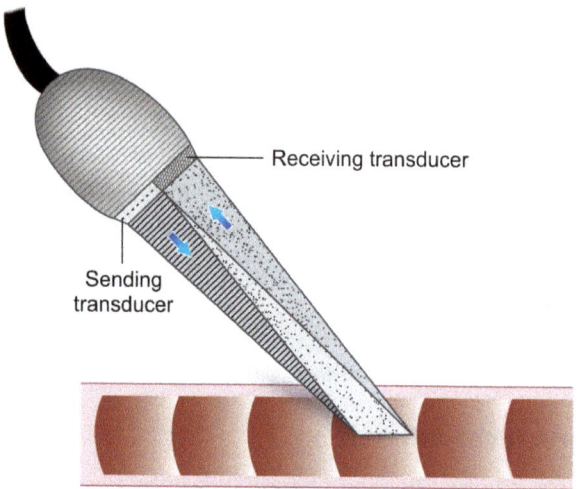

**Fig. 1.12:** Diagram of a pulsed-Doppler transducer demonstrating the direction of the transmitted sound beam toward the flow of blood and the receiving sound beam back to the transducer.

returns at a different frequency. The speed (velocity) of the moving structure can be calculated from this frequency shift **(Fig. 1.13)**. The returning frequency will be increased if flow is toward the sound source (transducer) and will be decreased if flow is away from the sound source.

## *Clinical Correlation*

The Doppler effect is helpful in localizing blood vessels and determining optimal sites for velocity measurements. Veins typically have a low-pitched hum, whereas arteries have an alternating pattern with a high-pitched systolic component and a low-pitched diastolic component.

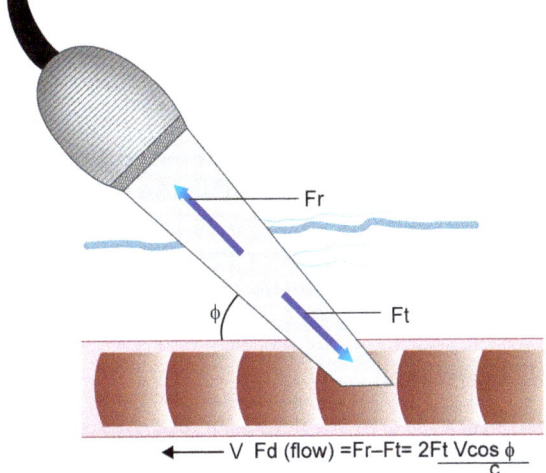

**Fig. 1.13:** Diagram showing the components of the Doppler equation. φ, angle of insonation of the vessel; c, speed of sound in tissue (–1,540 m/ sec). (Fr: return frequency; Ft: sending frequency; V: blood flow velocity).

## Continuous-wave Doppler

The sound beam is continuously emitted from one transducer crystal and is received by the second. Both transducers are encased in one housing.
- *Dedicated continues-wave (CVV) Doppler pencil probes.*
- Imaging CW Doppler.

### Clinical Correlation

Vascular surgeons use CW Doppler to check for the presence or absence of flow in superficial arteries. CW Doppler is also sometimes used to monitor umbilical artery flow. Because the cord lies in the amniotic fluid, no other confusing vessels are within the ultrasonic beam.

## Pulsed Doppler

A Doppler sound beam is sent and received (pulsed) over a short period of time. Because the time that the Doppler signal takes to reach the target can be converted to distance, the depth of the site sampled is known.

The pulsed sound beam is "gated." Only those signals from a vessel at a known depth are displayed and analyzed.

### Clinical Correlation

Pulsed Doppler is used to detect the presence of blood flow in a select vessel at a given depth when there are several vessels within the ultrasonic beam. Clots can appear echo-free, so a real time image may erroneously appear to show a normal vessel even if it is occluded. Doppler will detect no flow. Flow from other vessels outside the region of the gate is not analyzed because only the gated area is examined.

## Flow Direction

The direction of blood flow can be discovered by assessing whether the frequency of the returning signal is above or below the baseline in a suspect vessel. Flow toward the transducer is traditionally displayed above the baseline, and flow' away from the transducer is shown below the baseline.

### Clinical Correlation

Flow in the portal vein is sometimes reversed when pressure in the liver increases in portal hypertension; flow away from the liver is known as *hepatofugal* and indicates that the portal pressure is so high that flow has been reversed. A memory aid that some sonographers find useful to remember this often confusing terminology, is "fugitives flee." Flow toward the liver is known as *hepatopetal*. Flow direction analysis allows the diagnosis of the abnormal hepatofugal flow.

## Flow Pattern

The pattern of flow can be assessed with Doppler ultrasound. Typically, a vein shows a continuous rhythmic flow in diastole and systole and emits a lower pitched signal than does arterial flow. Arterial flow has an alternating high-pitched systolic peak and a much lower diastolic level.

### Clinical Correlation

Veins may be confused with arteries in real time.

## Flow Velocity

The velocity of blood flow can be deduced from the arterial waveform (**Fig. 1.14**). If the peak systolic flow frequency and the angle at which the beam intersects the vessel are known, a simple formula allows the calculation of velocity (**Fig. 1.13**). The velocity calculation formula is only accurate if the angle of the Doppler beam to the interrogated vessel is less than 60 degrees.

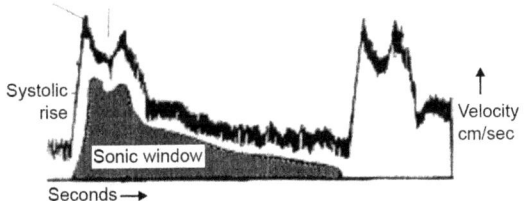

**Fig. 1.14:** Diagram of an arterial spectral waveform in a low resistance bed.

*Clinical Correlation*

Velocity is an important factor in calculating the severity of carotid stenosis. Generally, the more severe the stenosis is, the greater the velocity through the narrowed vessel will be. As the vessel becomes critically occluded, however, flow velocity will diminish.

## Low- versus High-resistance Flow

Doppler flow analysis allows the detection of two types of arterial flow: a high-resistance (**Fig. 1.15**) and a low-resistance pattern.

The high-resistance pattern has a high systolic peak and a low diastolic flow.

Low-resistance arterial systems demonstrate a biphasic systolic peak and a relatively high level of flow in diastole.

Resistance index (RI) is commonly calculated by the following formula:

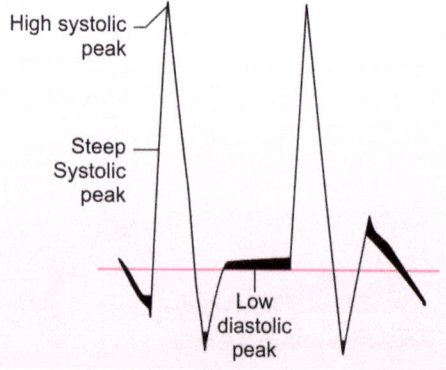

**Fig. 1.15:** Diagram of an arterial spectral waveform in a high resistance bed.

$$RI = \frac{\text{(Systolic velocity - Diastolic velocity)}}{\text{(Systolic velocity)}}$$

An alternative technique, known as the *pulsatility index* (PI), evaluates the diastolic flow in a different fashion. A cursor is run along the superior aspect of the systolic and diastolic flow envelope, and the mean is calculated by the system.

PI = (Systolic velocity - Mean flow)/(Systolic velocity)

In obstetrics, the A/B or systolic-diastolic (SID) ratio is commonly used:

$$SID = A/B = \frac{\text{(Peak systolic velocity)}}{\text{(End-diastolic velocity)}}$$

All three of these parameters (RI, PI, and SID ratio) are just different mathematical constructs that attempt to estimate the relative difference in flow velocity between systole and diastole.

### Clinical Correlation

If a high-resistance pattern is seen where there is normally a low-resistance appearance, such as in the common carotid or renal artery, vessel narrowing is present. Quantifying the severity of the resistance may help in clinical management.

A high-resistance pattern is usually seen in the vessel supplying the ovaries in the proliferative phase of the cycle.

If a low resistance pattern (RI < 0.4) is seen within an ovarian mass, carcinoma is more likely.

## Flow Pattern within a Vessel (Laminar Flow)

In a normal vessel, the velocity of blood is highest in the center of a vessel and is lowest closer to the wall. This condition is termed *laminar flow*. When there is a wall irregularity or if the artery is angled, the flow is distorted and may be greatest when it is closest to the vessel wall. Stenosis markedly increases the flow velocity—through an area of narrowing, whereas vessel dilatation decreases the speed of flow.

*Clinical Correlation*

To accurately measure the flow velocity in a tortuous carotid artery, place the sample volume (the area that is gated) at the center of the highest flow. Listening to the audible signal is useful in determining the site for optimal measurement. A high-grade stenosis will have a shrill, chirping sound.

## Flow Distortion

Normal laminar flow at and immediately beyond an area of wall irregularity or stenosis is disturbed, resulting in abnormal spectral waveforms. Flow distortion (nonlaminar) is characterized by high velocities in both systole and diastole. The presence of many echoes within the sonic window is termed *spectral broadening* and may indicate considerable flow disturbance.

*Clinical Correlation*

Flow disturbance in an artery such as the carotid may indicate pathologic atheromatous changes.

## Flow Changes beyond a Narrowed Area (Poststenotic Changes)

Poststenotic changes in arterial flow may be seen in the next few centimeters beyond a narrowed area. When there is severe stenosis, the systolic peak in the poststenotic area will be lower (more rounded) with lower velocities throughout diastole. The acceleration slope of the systolic peaks (peak systole) will be diminished. This pattern is known as the *tardus et parvus* abnormality. In less severe obstruction, the spectral waveform may resume the normal high- or low-resistance flow appropriate for that artery.

### Clinical Correlation

Detecting a poststenotic pattern is particularly valuable in evaluating the renal arteries because the usual site of stenosis, adjacent to the aorta, is rarely seen owing to the presence of bowel gas. Poststenotic changes may also be seen in the common carotid artery when the stenosis involves the origin of the common carotid. The waveform of the other common carotid should be evaluated for comparison. Large calcified plaques may obscure the area of stenosis, so one may be dependent on poststenotic changes to determine the severity of narrowing.

## Flow Volume

The flow volume through a given vessel can be roughly estimated if the velocity of flow and the vessel diameter are known.

### Clinical Correlation

The calculation of flow volume is important in situations in which a low level of flow is associated with inadequate function, e.g. penile arterial flow.

## Aliasing

If there is a marked frequency shift with a high measured velocity, the signal may return after the next pulse has started. This condition is called *aliasing*.

To compensate for aliasing, increase the velocity range (PRF). Lowering the baseline may also prevent aliasing.

*Clinical Correlation*

If aliasing is present, the peak signal will be inaccurately measured as lower than it really is, and the severity of the stenosis will be incorrectly measured.

## Color Flow Imaging

Color flow assigns different hues to the red blood cells in a vessel depending on their velocities and the direction of the blood flow relative to the transducer. This allocation is based on the Doppler principle.

*Clinical Correlation*

The site of maximum flow can be visualized quickly so that the pulsed Doppler gate can be inserted where the flow is highest.

## Color Flow Display and Direction within a Vessel

In most systems, flow toward the transducer is allocated red, and flow away from the transducer is allocated blue. The flow velocity is displayed with faster velocities in brighter colors and slower velocities in darker colors. The fastest velocity may be displayed in yellow or white. Turbulent flow will demonstrate a mixture of colors.

As with pulsed Doppler, optimal images are only obtained at an oblique angle. If a vessel runs a straight course, flow at 90 degrees to the color box will not be displayed. The angle of

Basics in Ultrasonography

the color box region of interest (ROI) can be adjusted to the left or right when linear steering is available; otherwise, the probe can be manually angled to provide the angle needed to receive the returning signals.

### Clinical Correlation

Soft plaque may be missed on gray scale but a flow void will be seen using color flow. Sometimes, soft plaques may show no changes on grayscale. Once correct color allocation has been made, normal vessels will fill with color.

## Knobology: Doppler and Color Flow

### Range Gate Cursor (Sample Volume)

The Doppler sample volume is displayed on the B-scan image. This cursor, which may be presented as a box or two parallel bars, indicates the depth and area from which the Doppler signal is obtained.

### Region of Interest

This box is used to restrict the color display of a blood flow image and to eliminate an unnecessary display of color.

### Inversion and Direction of Flow and Its Relation to Baseline (Doppler)

When blood flow is moving toward the transducer, sound waves of high frequency are reflected, and positive signals are seen above the baseline. Blood cells that are moving away from the transducer appear as negative signals below the baseline. Both veins and arteries can show flow in either direction because interpreting flow direction depends on the angle of the vessel to the transducer.

## Color Inversion

As in spectral Doppler, the display of color is dependent on the angle of the flow to the transducer.

## Color Flow Baseline

Blood flow toward the transducer will be shown within the measurable range of colors above the color bar baseline. Blood flow away from the probe will be displayed in the range of colors below the baseline.

## Velocity Scale/Velocity Range/PRF (Doppler)

The range of velocities that can be seen in the spectral display is determined by the PRF value. Higher velocity vessels (e.g. carotid) requires a high PRF; therefore, the velocity range should be increased.

## PRF (Color Flow)

The range of velocities used in color flow is lower compared to the spectral waveform because the average Doppler shift frequency is displayed rather than the peak velocity. Depending on the color map used, lower PRF values may present a shift to a different color, representing a slightly higher velocity flow (i.e. white or yellow).

## Sweep Speed (Doppler Only)

The rate at which the spectral information is displayed can be adjusted using the sweep speed controls. A slow speed (e.g. 25 mm/sec), a moderate speed (e.g. 50 mm/sec), or a fast speed (e.g. 100 mm/sec) can be selected.

## Wall Filter (Doppler)

Blood flow signals that are not wanted can be eliminated by using the wall filter.

## Filter (Color Flow)

A phenomenon called *color flash,* caused by cardiac or peristaltic motion or by transducer movement, produces a flash of spurious color in an area where there is no real flow. The area of interest can be concealed by the flash artifact.

## Gain (Doppler and Color Flow)

The gain controls alter the spectral waveform and the color flow image. Inadequate gain results in an image in which the vessel is incompletely filled with color or in which no spectral Doppler signal can be obtained in areas of slow flow.

## Angle Correct Bar (Flow Vector)

An angle correct bar is situated within the range gate cursor. This bar should be aligned with the direction of blood flow. The angle created by the insonating ultrasound beam and this bar must be known if the flow velocity is to be deduced from the frequency of the returning Doppler signal. The angle should be less than 60 degrees.

## Power Doppler

Power Doppler utilizes the amplitude of the Doppler signal to generate the ultrasound image. Areas with high concentrations of blood cells will appear in brighter colors while lower concentrations of blood cells will appear in darker colors. This technique is more sensitive for subtle flow than is conventional color flow Doppler. Power Doppler typically does not provide any directional information and is particularly useful for evaluating the presence of flow or low flow in small or subtle vessels (e.g., ovarian masses).

## Audio Volume

The Doppler sound will be heard from the built-in speakers. Usually, there are independent speakers for both forward and reverse flow. The control varies the volume of the Doppler sound.

## Cursor Movement Control

The cursor (range gate cursor and ROI) movement can be manipulated by means of a trackball or a joystick.

## Measurements

The standard measurement unit used in displaying the spectral waveform is velocity (m/sec or cm/sec). When dealing with a high grade stenosis, obtain maximum velocities at and just beyond the area of lumen narrowing.

# Pitfalls

## Incorrect Angle

A waveform that appears to indicate a distal obstruction is displayed in a vessel; however, no plaque is seen in the vessel.

### Correction Technique

Check the position of the ultrasound beam relation to the direction of flow. If the angle greater than 60 degrees, then the velocity is not being accurately calculated, and an abnormal waveform is created.

## Little or No Doppler Signal in an Artery

The spectral waveform shows apparent low systolic flow and minimal diastolic flow. This may be because of:
- There may be a severe obstruction proximal to this area and in an area too difficult to evaluate with the ultrasound beam (e.g., origin of the common carotid artery)
- This patient may have diminished cardiac output
- The sample volume (gate) may not be placed where maximum flow is present
- The sample volume is too large for the small amount of flow
- The wall filters level is set too high.

### Correction Technique

- Do not depend solely on the visualization of the vessel
- Color flow highlights the higher velocities in the artery and helps in gate placement, but a keen ear is more sensitive
- A higher velocity may be evident as the sound beam is angled slightly off the center of the stream
- *A larger sample size may be needed when scanning to locate the site of flow, but to obtain a more precise flow measurement within an artery, decrease the gate size*
- The wall filter *should be set at the lowest setting that does not introduce artifacts, especially when scanning a vein (a low-flow state)*

Try the following maneuvers before giving up:
- Change to another acoustic window or different incident angle
- Open up the gate setting
- Lower the velocity' range

- Use a lower frequency transducer. The patient may be too obese for a higher frequency transducer.

## A High-resistance Waveform in a Low-resistance Bed

### Explanation

There may be soft plaque distal to this area. If the B-scan gain is too low, soft plaque may be missed. Use color flow to outline the true patent lumen.

## Aliasing

A tight stenosis causes such high velocities at the site of flow and immediately distal to the narrowed area that flow is seen above the baseline and at the lower edge of the spectral display. When color is used, there may be peaks of color from the other end of the spectrum. A chirping sound may be heard as you angle through the stenotic area.

This may be due to the fact that, the velocity is so high that the signal wraps around itself, and peak velocities are displayed below the baseline. This problem arises because the selected PRF is too low to accurately pick up the high velocities that are occurring.

### Correction Techniques

- Place the baseline at its lowest site to allow the systolic peaks to be displayed
- Increase the PRF (velocity range)
- Some units allow the B-scan image to be frozen while the Doppler signal is obtained. This will also widen the measurable velocity range

- Increase the Doppler angle, but do not exceed 60 degrees
- Decrease the insonating frequency. Most units offer a choice of several Doppler frequencies for each transducer. Otherwise, change to a lower frequency transducer
- Change to CW (not widely available on most current machines).

## Inadequate Venous Signal

Venous flow is difficult to detect even when the vessel is clearly demonstrated. This may be due to:
- There may be little venous flow at rest
- The vein may be compressed by patient position
- The B-scan gain may be too low to demonstrate the clot within the vein.

### Correction Technique

- Respiration affects venous flow. With inspiration and the descent of the diaphragm, pressure increases in the abdomen. Ask the patient to perform a Valsalva maneuver. As the breath is released, venous flow increases, and the venous signal will become more pronounced
- Ask the patient to flex the leg slightly and re-evaluate. Use color flow' in these instances to accentuate subtle flow
- Increase the gain and apply gentle compression to see if the vein collapses.

## Audible Signal but Vessel not Seen

A venous signal can be heard, but a patent vessel cannot be visualized.

The vein may be subtotally occluded, or the presence of adjacent collaterals may cause the audible signal.

## Correction Technique

Color flow will demonstrate the smaller collateral vessels as well as a small amount of residual flow in an almost occluded vessel.

## Spectral Broadening

Apparent spectral broadening may be caused by too much gain or by scanning too close to the vessel wall, picking up lower velocities.

### Correction Technique

Make sure the supposed spectral broadening reflects true pathology and is not just noise by comparing it to an area known to be normal.

## A Flickering Image

Sometimes, it is difficult to evaluate color flow when obtaining a pulsed Doppler signal because the image flickers.

A large amount of data is being processed to generate the image for each frame of information when obtaining the Doppler signal or color flow. Therefore, the frame rate is lowered, and a flicker may occur.

### Correction Technique

To reduce this flicker, evaluate one mode at a time (e.g. use color flow only) or reduce the width of the color flow box.

## Color Misregistration Artifact (Color Flash)

If the transducer is rapidly moved, a flash of color related to transducer movement and not to vascular flow may develop.

## Correction Technique

Use the filter to reduce noise and move the transducer slowly, using caution not to remove real vascular flow from the image.

## Tissue Vibration or Transmitted Pulsation

In the region of a highly pulsatile structure such as an artery, neighboring structures may move, causing some color artifact in the surrounding tissues.

## Correction Technique

Scan from a different axis if possible.

## Active Peristalsis

Active peristalsis may induce a color flow artifact.

## Undue Color Gain

The outline of vessels may be misregistered owing to excessive gain, so the flow appears to fill in some of the surrounding tissues (color bleed).

## Correction Technique

Decrease gain so the color image corresponds to the vessel outline.

# EQUIPMENT CARE AND QUALITY CONTROL

Ultrasound systems are precision instruments that require careful handling and regular maintenance to ensure optimum performance.

## Preventive Maintenance

- Liquids other than contact gel should not be stored on the equipment
- The hand used to adjust control settings should be kept clean to ensure that contact gel does not affect the trackball or other functions
- Cables and transducers should be visually inspected for worn areas or cracks
- Careless placement of the transducer and cable on the machine can cause cable damage
- Transducers should be placed in proper holders to avoid stress on cables
- When taking ultrasound equipment to wards, it should be moved carefully to avoid sudden impact, which may dislodge printed circuit boards from their connectors, resulting in failure of operation
- Many ultrasound systems have cooling fans with overlying air filters to prevent deposition of dust and particles on circuit boards within the unit. These should be cleaned periodically (weekly), especially if used in carpeted areas
- Error messages should be noted and recorded for referral to service personnel.

## Transducer Care

Transducers are delicate instruments and require careful handling. Transducers that have been dropped or treated roughly may have "dead" elements that no longer transmit or receive signals (due to debonding of electrodes from crystal elements).

Each time a transducer is removed from its cradle, ensure that the transducer cable is not snagged on part of

# Basics in Ultrasonography

the ultrasound system (such as the wheel support). The compromised length of cable may result in the transducer being pulled out of the hand as it is moved toward the patient.

Transducers should be cleaned after each patient with an alcohol sponge or transducer disinfectant, particularly if the patient has an open wound or a skin problem. Plastic freezer bags are an inexpensive means of covering the transducer to avoid contact with open wounds and to avoid contamination. Some transducers can be immersed in Cidex up to the handle for sterilization. Approximately 10 minutes of immersion is required for adequate sterilization.

Use a commercial water-soluble coupling gel to ensure good acoustic contact between the transducer and patient. Thick, high-viscosity gels are desirable when scanning the patient in an erect position because they don't slide off easily. Thicker gels are also helpful for obstetric patients with large abdomens.

Use disposable gloves when scanning a patient to avoid the risk of infection. Spread the gel around the abdomen with the transducer rather than by hand. Do not handle the controls with gel on your hand or glove.

## Quality Assurance

Quality assurance tests may be tedious to perform but are worthwhile because it may be difficult or even impossible to detect calibration and measurement distortions from examination of the images alone. Clearly, major clinical problems may result if erroneous measurement data are produced. Quality assurance checks should be performed on a quarterly basis with most systems or more often if a problem a suspected, e.g., if a transducer has been dropped or measurements are consistently higher or lower than expected.

## Quality Control Tests

The standard tests performed to ensure that the system is working satisfactorily are:
- Aspect ratio and calibration tests
- Resolution tests (both axial and lateral)
- A comparative power output test that equates to a depth of penetration measurement.

All these tests are performed on a tissue-equivalent phantom.

## Aspect Ratio and Calibration Test

The aspect ratio and calibration test measures whether distances are accurate in both directions—horizontal and vertical directions and whether these measurements are displayed accurately on a hard-copy device transducer.

## Resolution

Axial and lateral resolution capability can be determined using closely spaced pins in a phantom.

## Comparative Power Output

The test for comparative power output determines whether the sound beam emitted by the transducer can reach a depth adequate to see deep structures. The test is performed at full power output, and the time gain compensation is set at maximum at the area of depth visualization. The comparative power output can be calculated as follows:

Attenuation factor (0.7) × Depth (7.35) × Transducer frequency (5) = 25.725 dB

This number is recorded in the quality control logbook as the output for this transducer using this phantom. Repeat tests should give the same result. For the comparison of results to be valid, all settings must be the same each time the test is undertaken. This is a useful test to see whether transmitter and/or receiver characteristics are changing over time.

## Malfunction

Modem ultrasound systems are very reliable but occasionally can malfunction, resulting in disruption of images.

This is rare in modem systems, but when it occurs, it is usually obvious with clear disruption of the images.

The disruption may relate to circuitry for a specific transducer, so the equipment may still be usable with different transducers until the problem can be rectified. Occasionally, a transducer that has been selected may not initialize correctly, or its connection to the ultrasound system may be fault, but can be corrected by disconnecting and reconnecting the transducer so that it re-initializes.

Software errors occasionally occur and can often be rectified by switching the ultrasound unit off and on again, allowing the system to reboot. It may be necessary to wait 30 seconds before switching the system on again to allow time for correction of the software error.

## MALPRACTICE AND ULTRASOUND

## Causes of Malpractice

Legally malpractice as it relates to ultrasound comes in two forms:
1. *Battery injury:* The patient is injured during the examination by assault or inadequate care (e.g., falls off the table). Failure to obtain informed consent is another type of "battery" injury.

2. *Negligence:* The examination is performed in a fashion that is "below the standard of care."

*Standard of care* is defined as the way in which a "reasonable and prudent" physician or sonographer would act under the same circumstances. In our court system, the standard of care is established in several inherent ways:
- Expert witnesses testify as to the standard of care
- Guidelines such as the American Institute of Ultrasound in Medicine (AIUM) "Practice Guidelines for the Performance of an Antepartum Obstetric Ultrasound Examination" or American Congress of Obstetricians and Gynecologists technical bulletins set national standards. There are no such laid down in our country
- Local hospital, radiology, or obstetric department policy statements also set the standard of care.

## Responsibilities of the Physician or Sonographer Reporting the Study

- The physician or sonographer reporting the study is required to accurately describe the findings on the examination, including pertinent negative findings with a clinical conclusion about the presence or absence of an abnormality
- Suggestions about additional procedures or follow-up studies may be required
- Problems in the performance of the study, such as obesity or suboptimal patient position, should be covered in the narrative portion of the report
- A preliminary report is not considered legally hazardous as long as the sonographer does not attempt to make a diagnosis

- If a sonographer is working for a sonologist, the sonographer is not responsible for errors in the study, provided that the study is performed according to standards set by the sonologist, even if the study is of poor quality
- The sonographer is not liable if he or she uses a technique that creates an image that looks like pathology but is not
- Some examples of misleading findings or wrong techniques that are not the sonographers legal responsibility if uncorrected by the sonologist are the following:
    - Pseudohydronephrosis as the result of a full urinary bladder
    - Sludge-filled gallbladder due to an overgained image
    - Not following up on a pathologic finding, such as missing hydronephrosis with a pelvic mass
    - Missing a pancreatic mass by not trying different scanning techniques, such as erect scanning or having the patient drink to fill the stomach to create an acoustic window
    - Missing stones in the gallbladder or kidneys due to a failure to use a high-frequency transducer.

Although the sonographer is not held legally responsible for these errors, there is still the moral and ethical element to consider.

## Responsibilities of the Physician or Sonographer Performing the Examination

- The primary responsibility is to perform a comprehensive examination that conforms to the national standards
- One should care for the patient and make sure that the patient comes to no harm by rough treatment or carelessness
- Confidentiality must be observed.

Some examples of situations in which a sonographer is liable are:
- *Physically molesting the patient*
- *Letting a patient fall, causing injury*
- *Giving the patient or accompanying doctor a wrong diagnosis*
- *Revealing confidential information about the contents of the sonogram* or disclosing any information that has adverse effects on the patient

## Legally Hazardous Situations

### Emergency Studies

Emergency ultrasound studies often modify clinical management from conservative to aggressive, and because any management changes hinge on the sonographic findings, the examination may be legally hazardous.

Litigation is common when a wrong diagnosis leads to immediate consequences.

Some examples of emergency situations often followed by litigation are as follows:
- *Failure to recognize ectopic pregnancy;* Few ectopic pregnancies now require immediate surgery because many are now treated with methotrexate. This has created a new risk: misdiagnosis of a normal pregnancy as an ectopic pregnancy with subsequent methotrexate treatment with survival of a deformed but viable intrauterine pregnancy
- *Failure to diagnose ovarian torsion*
- *Misdiagnosis of fetal death:* Wrongly diagnosing fetal death with the subsequent delivery of a live but damaged infant can occur

- *Failure to diagnose abruptio placenta*
- *Failure to diagnose a fetal anomaly:* Fetal abnormalities are a common cause of litigation because the monetary award for a missed anomaly is so large. Litigation related to obstetric ultrasound is many times more frequent than for all other types of ultrasound combined
- The common missed fetal abnormalities resulting in litigation are as follows:
    - Missed spina bifida
    - Hypoplastic left heart syndrome
    - Absent limb or limbs
    - Down syndrome signs
    - Hydrocephalus.

Often, the litigation concerns a basic level obstetric study in which there is a possibility of an abnormality and no recommendation is made for referral for a targeted or referral study to be performed at a specialized center.

## Failure to Diagnose Major Obstetric Findings

Some obstetric ultrasound findings that have been overlooked and that have serious consequences to pregnancy management are as follows:

- *Twins or triplets:* Failure to diagnose twins or triplets can lead to severe long-term disability if the presence of twins is first discovered at delivery.
- *Unrecognized placenta previa* during a sonographic examination may lead to a major bleed at delivery.
- *Breast cancer that is misdiagnosed as merely a breast cyst:* Failure to diagnose breast cancer is the most common cause of imaging litigation. Most suits relate to mammography, but breast cancer ultrasound cases are occurring increasingly.

## Substandard Reporting of the Ultrasound Study

- *Dating an obstetric study in the third trimester:* The range of possible dates for a series of obstetric measurements such as the biparietal diameter, head circumference, femur length, and abdominal circumference in the third trimester is ± three to four weeks, so accurate dating if the patient presents in the third trimester is not possible. This error is so well known that the obstetrician and radiologist share responsibility if delivery is performed before fetal viability under these circumstances
- *Dating or weight estimation with unsatisfactory measurement data:* It is not always possible to obtain a quality abdominal circumference or fetal head measurements with an unusual fetal position. Problems of this type should be noted in the report. Not reporting these problems may result in wrong clinical decisions about delivery or the presence of intrauterine growth restriction (IUGR)
- *Failure to compare the dates or weight on the current examination with earlier sonographic studies* may mean a failure to diagnose IUGR. Data from earlier sonograms should be obtained if later examinations are performed at another facility.

## Tardy Reporting

- Delayed reporting of an ultrasound study or delayed transmission of an ultrasound report to the referring doctor can lead to litigation.

- Findings that change management, such as the discovery of an ectopic pregnancy or a low biophysical profile score of 0 to 2, require immediate notification to the managing physician.
- Some examples of serious consequences of a delayed report are as follows:
  - *Failure to relay a report of a placenta previa* resulted in the loss of the pregnancy in a patient with heavy vaginal bleeding
  - *Two week delay in transmitting a report of IUGR* resulting in the loss of that pregnancy.

Failure to Perform an Appropriate Ultrasound Study when a Patient Presents with a Family History of a Malformation Or a Drug History predisposing to a Malformation.

A common indication of an ultrasound study is a family history of fetal malformations or when the patient is taking drugs like valproic acid, that causes the fetal malformations. Specific views of potential malformations such as the lumbar spine with valproic acid or the face with a family history of cleft lip and palate, need to be obtained and reported.

## Interventional Guidance Problems

Amniocentesis for chromosomal abnormality or to establish fetal lung maturity is still commonly performed and is standardly performed under ultrasound guidance. Suits related to fetal damage or fetal death due to the procedure still occur. Documentation of the amniocentesis site and of fetal viability after the procedure and a written report of the way in which the procedure was performed are helpful in avoiding litigation and defending complaints. By convention, only two passes are made if aspiration of amniotic fluid is unsuccessful.

## MALPRACTICE INSURANCE: WHO NEEDS IT?

Any sonographer performing freelance work should invest in malpractice insurance. Sonographers employed by a hospital or other institution do not generally need to purchase insurance because they are covered by the hospital's or clinic's policy.

# CHAPTER 2

# Training

The practice of ultrasound and the use of diagnostic and interventional ultrasound is like a stethoscope to the gynecologist today. It is impossible to even conceive a gynecology diagnostic unit without ultrasound.

## AIMS OF THE TRAINING SCHEDULE

- Ability to visualize in two-dimensional image and a three-dimensional structure.
- Hand-eye coordination.
- Supervision is essential.
- Level of training depending on competence.

## REQUIRED SKILLS

The trainee should be able to identify:
- Normal pelvic anatomy
- Uterine size and endometrial thickness
- Measurement of ovaries
- Pelvic tumors, e.g. fibroids, cysts hydrosalpinx
- Peritoneal fluid
- Intrauterine contraceptive devices.

## THEORETICAL TRAINING PROGRAM

It helps the trainee to understand and be able to discuss the following.

# Basic Principles of Medical Ultrasound

- The relevant principles of acoustics, attenuation, absorption, reflection, speed to sound
- The effect on tissues of pulsed and continuous-wave ultrasound beams: biological effects, thermal and non-thermal
- Basic operating principles of medical instruments:
    - Pulse echo, scanning principles and 3D
    - Pulse echo instruments, including linear array, curvilinear, mechanical sector, transvaginal and rectal scanners
    - Velocity imaging and recording:
        ⇒ Doppler principle
        - Continuous wave
        - Pulse wave
        - Color flow mapping
        - Power Doppler
        ⇒ Color velocity imaging
        ⇒ Pitfalls, artifacts
    - Data acquisition
    - Signal processing (may be given in practical demonstration):
        ⇒ Gray scale
        ⇒ Time gain compensation
        ⇒ Dynamic range
        ⇒ Dynamic focus
        ⇒ Gain compensation, acoustic output relationship (may be given in practical demonstration)
    - Artefacts, interpretation and avoidance
        ⇒ Reverberation ⇒ Side lobes
        ⇒ Edge effects ⇒ Registration
        ⇒ Shadowing ⇒ Enhancement

- Measuring systems
  - ⇒ Linear, circumference, area and volume
  - ⇒ Doppler ultrasound—flow, velocity spectrum analysis
- Imaging recording, storage and analysis
- Interpretation of acoustic output information and its clinical relevance.

## GYNECOLOGICAL ULTRASOUND

- Normal pelvic anatomy
  - Uterus
    - ⇒ Uterine size, position, shape and movement
    - ⇒ Cyclical morphological changes in the endometrium
    - ⇒ Measurement of endometrial thickness
  - Ovaries
    - ⇒ Size, position, shape and measurement
    - ⇒ Cyclical morphological changes
    - ⇒ Measurement of follicles and corpus luteum
    - ⇒ Assessment of peritoneal fluid.
- Gynecological complications
  - Uterus
    - ⇒ Fibroids    ⇒ Adenomyosis
    - ⇒ Endometrial hyperplasia
    - ⇒ Endometrial cancer   ⇒ Polyps
    - ⇒ Location of intrauterine contraceptive device.
  - Tubes
    - ⇒ Hydrosalpinx and other abnormalities of the fallopian tubes.
  - Ovaries
    - ⇒ Cysts; benign and malignant, morphological scoring systems

- ⇒ Endometriosis
- ⇒ Ovarian carcinoma
- ⇒ Differential diagnosis of pelvic masses
- Infertility
  - Monitoring of follicular development in spontaneous and stimulated cycles
    - ⇒ Diagnosis of hyperstimulation syndrome
    - ⇒ Diagnosis of polycystic ovaries
    - ⇒ Sonosalpingography
- Invasive procedures
  - Oocyte retrieval
  - Injection of ovarian cysts
  - Aspiration of ovarian cysts
  - Drainage of pelvic abscesses
  - Extraction of intrauterine contraceptive device
- Doppler in gynecology
  - Infertility and oncology.

## PRACTICAL TRAINING

### Requirement Skills

- The trainee should be able to identify gynecological problems by transvaginal and transabdominal ultrasound.
- Normal pelvic anatomy
- Uterine size and endometrial thickness
- Measurement of ovaries
- Pelvic tumors, e.g. fibroids, cysts, hydrosalpinx
- Peritoneal fluid
- Intrauterine contraceptive devices.

# CHAPTER 3

# Introduction

## FILLING UP OF FORMS

Maintain a form for further follow-up in your clinic. One never knows when the information is required.
The routine information required in these forms is:
- Name
- Age
- Address
- Telephone number
- Referred by.

## RELEVANT HISTORY

Always spend few minutes with your patient to take the details of the history. Gives confidence to the patient and you get your perspective of what all to expect.
The history to be taken routinely is:
- Symptoms and their details. Check for menstrual history (duration and regularity). Check in the patient's language about menorrhagia, metrorrhagia, menometrorrhagia, intermenstrual spotting, dyspareunia, pain lower abdomen, pain in the lower back and any urinary and lower complaints.
- Check duration and cyclicity of symptoms.
- Any ultrasound done previously. Check the records carefully.

- Last menstrual period.
- Any tests done and their reports.
- Referring doctors requisition slip.

## PREPARATION AND POSITIONING OF PATIENTS

- The patient need not be fasting unless and until an upper abdomen scan is also asked for.
- Make it a practice to have a full bladder for all gynecological ultrasounds. This will enable you to have a broader perspective and overview of all pelvic organs.
- The patient is almost always scanned supine with little jelly on the abdomen.
- Whenever, a transvaginal scan is asked for the bladder must be emptied immediately before the examination. It should be performed with the same respect for privacy and gentleness, as is with the placement of a speculum. Scanning is performed with the patient supine and with her thighs abducted and knees flexed. Elevation of the buttock may be necessary. The probe should be covered with a condom or sheath containing a small amount of gel. Additional gel should be placed on the outside of sheathed tip. The probe is inserted by a gentle push posteriorly toward the rectum while the patient relaxes. Four types of probe movements are required:
  - Pushing and pulling
  - Rotation
  - "Rocking" or upwards and downwards
  - Side-to-side or "Panning".

After removal of the transvaginal probe, the sheath is removed and the coupling gel is wiped off with a damp towel. The TV probe may be disinfected by Cidex.

# Introduction

## MACHINE AND TRANSDUCERS

- For a transabdominal scan, a 3.5–5.0 MHz transducer and for a transvaginal scan, a 5.0–8.0 MHz transducer is used.
- Basic controls of every machine are more or less the same. The placement of knobs is different for all machines. Check for the manual of your machine or somebody from the company can always come and explain you.

  The routine knobology is:
  - Patient's name and entry of last menstrual period after you select the obstetric mode.
  - Freeze
  - B, B+B, B+M or only M mode
  - Depth and focus
  - Overall gain
  - Time gain (TGC)
  - Comments on screen
  - Measurement (Set and Select) for linear, area and volume
  - Track ball or screen or joy stick to move the cursor
  - Color flow map, power Doppler, Doppler and 3D and 4D
  - After freezing the images these can be stored and a print taken on a camera, thermal printer or from a computer.

## REPORTING

In your reporting the salient features that require to be mentioned are:
- *Uterus:* Size, shape, mobility and probe tenderness.
- *Endometrium:* Thickness and morphology. Any focal abnormality to be mentioned with size and echo pattern.

- *Myometrium:* Echo pattern and presence of fibroids and their location.
- *Ovaries:* Size (all three dimensions with total volume) and echo pattern. Any abnormality to be mentioned in terms of size, echo pattern, walls and focal abnormalities within it.
- *Extra-ovarian adnexal areas:* Report whether any mass is delineated or not.
- *Free fluid* or fluid loculi in the pouch of Douglas or adnexa.

# CHAPTER 4

# Normal Anatomy of Female Pelvis

## UTERUS

- Pear shaped
- *Length:* 7 cm
- *Anteroposterior thickness:* 2.5 cm
- *Length of cavity:* 6 cm
- Body cervix ratio
  - *At birth:* 1:1
  - *Adult:* 2:1
- Corpus is divided into
  - *Isthmus:* Just above the internal Os
  - *Cornu:* At insertion of fallopian tube
- *Fundus:* Above the level of cornu

## CERVIX

- Constitutes the lower part of uterus
- *Total length:* 2.5–3 cm
- Divided into
  - Supravaginal cervix
  - Portio vaginalis
- Parts
  - External os

- Internal os
- Endocervical canal between the two
- Structure
  - Fibromuscular wall
  - Endocervical canal—columnar epithelium
  - Endocervix—stratified squamous epithelium
  - Glands—secrete mucus

## FALLOPIAN TUBES

- Length
  - About 10 cm
- Four parts
  1. Interstitial (narrowed) within the uterine cornu
  2. Isthmus (narrow) close to uterine cornu
  3. Ampullary (broader), thin walled lateral to isthmus
  4. Infundibulum (funnel shaped) ends in fimbriae
- Functions
  - Ovum pick up
  - Site of fertilization
  - Transport of fertilized ovum

## OVARIES

- Size
  - 3 × 2 cm
- Mesovarium (mesentery)
  - Posterior surface of broad ligament
- Ovarian ligament
  - Uterine cornu
- Infundibulopelvic ligament
  - Lateral pelvic wall.

**Figure 4.1** shows anatomy of female pelvis.

## Normal Anatomy of Female Pelvis

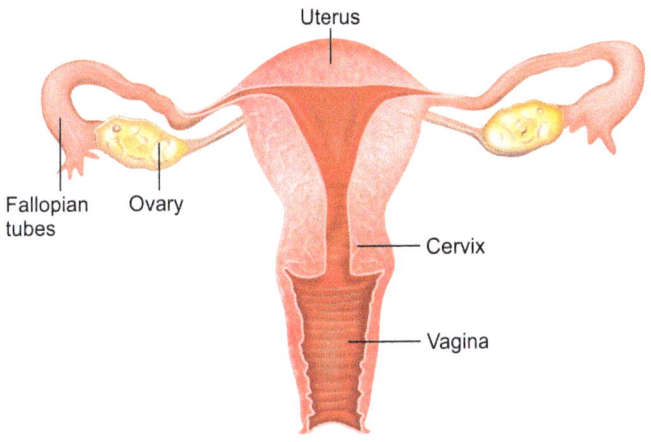

**Fig. 4.1:** Anatomy of female pelvis.

# CHAPTER 5

# Pelvic Sonography

## TRANSVAGINAL SONOGRAPHY

### Pelvic Sonography

Initial imaging tool of choice for assessing suspected gynecological disorders in patients of all ages.

#### Advantages

- Advantages are availability, low cost, lack of exposure to ionizing radiations and often the only imaging modality necessary for diagnosis of pelvic disease.
- Furthermore, is extremely useful in evaluation of urinary, gastrointestinal and musculoskeletal abnormalities that may mimic presentation of gynecologic disease.
- In most centers, the standard protocol begins with a transabdominal sonography (TAS) using a full urinary bladder (acoustic window) followed by transvaginal sonography (TVS) after emptying it and placing patient in lithotomy position.
- The two imaging modulates (TAS and TVS) are complementary, providing different diagnostic information.
- The TAS provides a wider field of view so a better visualization of superficial structures and large pelvic masses but has limited resolution.

- The TVS provides the probe to placed closer to the "target organs" providing better resolution, but limited field of view.
- The TVS is considered the optimal sonographic technique with highest diagnostic yield in female pelvis as it has the ability to use higher frequency probe providing the best anatomic details. An additional advantage is that, using the probe tip to assess pelvic structure for tenderness and localize it to the organ of concern.
- Not all patients are appropriate candidates for TVS.
- Transperineal, translabial and transrectal sonography are alternative approaches for imaging the female pelvic being mainly useful in the evaluation of the postmenopausal pelvic structures.

## *Indications*

- Evaluation of pelvic pain and pelvic masses.
- Evaluation of endocrine abnormalities (PCO).
- Evaluation of dysmenorrhea, amenorrhea, abnormal vaginal bleeding and delayed menses.
- Evaluation, monitoring and treatment of infertile patient.
- Evaluation of pelvic anatomy in a setting of limited clinical examination.
- Evaluation of suspected pelvic infection.
- Further, evaluation of the pelvic abnormality noted on another imaging study.
- Evaluation of congenital uterine and lower genital tract anomalies.
- Evaluation of excessive bleeding, pain or signs of infection after pelvic surgery, delivery, or abortion.
- Localization of an intrauterine contraceptive device.
- Screening for malignancy in high-risk patients.
- Evaluation of incontinence and pelvic organ prolapse.

- Evaluation of possible ectopic pregnancy.
- Evaluation of a first trimester gestation for viability, growth and abnormalities.
- Evaluation of the placenta, cervix and other pelvic structures in second and third trimester and also fatal anatomy.
- Guidance for interventional or surgical procedures.

## Contraindications

- The TVS must not be performed in patient who does not willingly give consent for the procedure.
- Not recommended in premenarchal or virgins.
- If a patient experiences anxiety or discomfort during insertion of probe terminate TVS and go for TAB. Patient may also be asked to insert the probe on her own.
- In postmenopausal women also, if they find it difficult to tolerate TVS, a transrectal, transperineal or translabial approach may be used.
- The TVS may also not very useful in evaluation of pelvic organ prolapse cervix and lower urinary tract.
- It is also contraindicated in some second and third trimester obstetric patents with active bleeding or rupture of membranes.
- The TVS examination may be compromised by a large/calcified leiomyoma in the lower uterus, large uterine size, fixation of the uterus to anterior abdominal wall after caesarean, positioning of the ovaries or other lesions high up in the pelvis beyond the field of view of TVS probe.
  - The TVS is also not preferred where a more panoramic view of the entire pelvis is required especially in cases of large pelvic mass or assessment and quantification of intra-abdominal disease.

# Protocols for Pelvic Sonography

Protocols can be tailored according to the specific clinical indication and there should be liberalization in using different protocols.

I. Standard protocol
   Complete TAS with full urinary bladder as acoustic window
   ↓
   TVS after emptying bladder

II. Alternate protocol
    TAB irrespective of fullness of bladder
    ↓
    VOID
    ↓
    TVS is performed

III. TVS with empty bladder
     ↓
     In case one/both ovary is not visible
     Incomplete visualization of large uterus or pelvic mass
     ↓
     TAS with empty/partially filled urinary bladder
     If examination is still incomplete
     ↓
     Ask the patient to fill the bladder
     ↓
     Repeat TAB

## PATIENT AND PROBE PREPARATION

- Highest possible frequency of transducer is used for better details of target organs.

- The TAS visualization of pelvic organs is limited by second attenuation due to anterior abdominal wall, subcutaneous and preperitoneal fat and also fat in mesentery and omentum.
- The TVS is performed using a probe of 7.5 MHz or higher frequency, taking advantage of placing the probe close to the pelvic organs with fewer intervening structures.
- The patient should immediately void before the TVS examination.
- A pertinent history should be elicited, rationale for performing TVS and how TVS will be performed must be explained to the patient.
- A verbal consent should be obtained.
- If a male sonologist is performing the scan, a female staff member should be present throughout the procedure.
- The patient should be laid comfortably in a lithotomy position and appropriately covered and draped and conducted in privacy.
- To prevent the spread of infection, the TVS probe should be appropriately disinfected using high level disinfections protocols provided by the manufacture's guide. Following disinfection, probe is wiped clean and a small amount of gel inside a probe covers. Care is taken to minimize air bubbles over the transducer face.

The probe tip should be lubricated with sterile, non-spermicidal gel.

The sonographer should wear sterile gloves while preparing the probe and performing the examination.

## IMAGING TECHNIQUE

- The patient, sonographer may introduce the TVS probe under real time monitoring.

- After insertion the probe must be positioned to optimize imaging of pelvic organs, by placing the probe in the anterior or lateral fornix and by application of gradually applying firm pressure against the vaginal wall.
- The orientation of the image is controlled by probe rotation and angulation.
- Perform a general pelvic survey by slowly sweeping the ultrasound beam in a long axis from midline through the adnexa continuing out to the pelvic side walls on each side.
- Probe is then rotated 90° counter clockwise into the short axis and beam is swept from the cervix to the fundus of the uterus.
- The probe is then angled to each side of the pelvis and scanning is performed sweeping both superiorly and inferiorly through each adnexal region.
- The probe can be advanced or withdrawn which will displace bowel and allow structures to be placed in the focal zone of the transducer.
- Normally, the pelvic structures must slide over one another with probe pressure. If the mobility is restricted it indicates adhesions.
- Visualization of the pelvic anatomy can be enhanced by applying pressure on the patient's anterior abdominal wall by the nonscanning hand or using a bimanual approach.
- After the survey, a set of static images is obtained, properly labeled and orientation of probe mentioned.
- The long axis TVS view is usually labeled the sagittal imaging plane and the short axis view as coronal/transverse.
- Imaging protocol includes:

- One/more static sagittal view of posterior cut-de-sac, cervix, midline uterus (AP dimension) parasagittal right and left uterine body, midline sagittal endometrial and right and left ovary.
- Coronal/transverse static images include posterior cut-de-sac, cervix, uterus at the fundal, mid-body, lower uterine segment and right and left ovary.
- Additionally, any disease must be assessed and appropriate additional images recorded.

# CHAPTER 6

# Normal Female Pelvis

Transabdominal and transvaginal scanning are two methods which complement each other and allow for a complete evaluation of the pelvic organs.

Evaluation of the normal female pelvis comprises of checking the pelvic viscera in detail comprises of:

## UTERUS

It is pear-shaped organ lies between urinary bladder anteriorly and rectum posteriorly.

## Size

Normal uterine size varies with age.

*Neonatal age*: Period between birth and fourth week after delivery. Neonatal uterus is relatively large due to increased levels of residual maternal hormones, has no isthmic part, with the body being larger than cervix.

*Infancy*: It is a time between four weeks and five years. In this period, uterus has a tubular shape, and at this time cervix is larger than corpus and it comprises two-thirds of whole uterine length, i.e. uterine body being smaller than the cervix **(Fig. 6.1)**.

*Childhood*: Period between two years of age and menarche uterine body again increases in size and acquired inverted pear-shape and increases longitudinally.

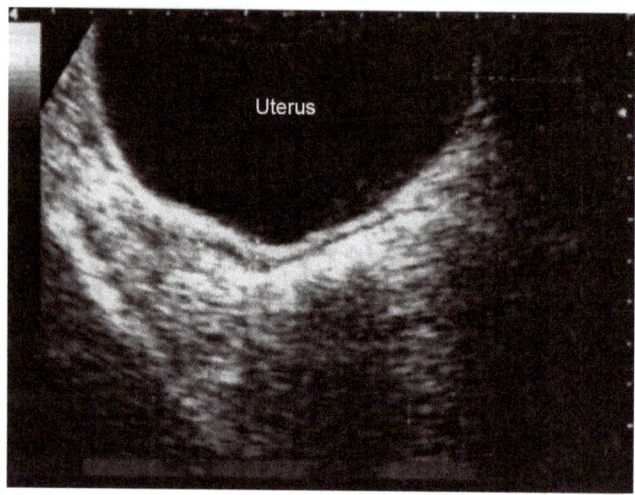

**Fig. 6.1:** Infantile uterus has a tubular shape with the uterine body being smaller than the cervix.

At puberty, i.e. in postmenarchal period, due to gradual increase of estrogen hormones, uterus grows faster and pear-shaped prominent.

During reproductive age group while uterus becomes two times bigger, with each pregnancy size of uterus increases by 1 cm. Size of uterus 7.5–9 cm × 2.5–4 cm × 4.5–5 cm **(Fig. 6.2)**.

In the postmenopausal uterus size starts to decrease due to reduced level of estrogen hormones and becomes 4.5 cm × 1.5 cm × 2.5 cm **(Fig. 6.3)**.

## DIVISIONS

Fundus, body (Corpus) and cervix **(Fig. 6.4)**. The body of the uterus is separated from the cervix by the isthmus at the level of the internal os **(Figs. 6.5 to 6.10)** and the angle of body of the uterus at the isthmus (flexion). The

Normal Female Pelvis

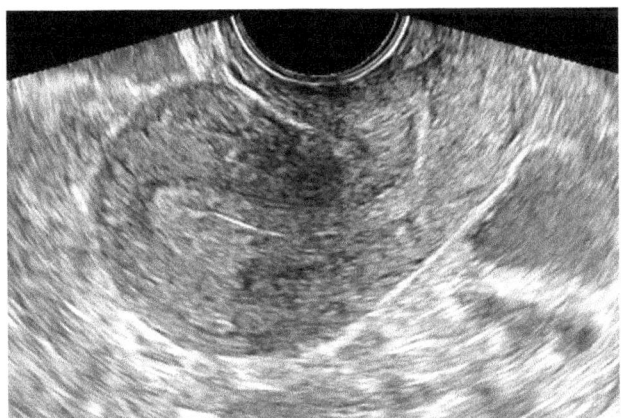

**Fig. 6.2:** In the postmenarchal period, the body is typically twice the size of the cervix. The dimensions of the normal uterus in women of childbearing age is 80 × 40 × 40 mm.

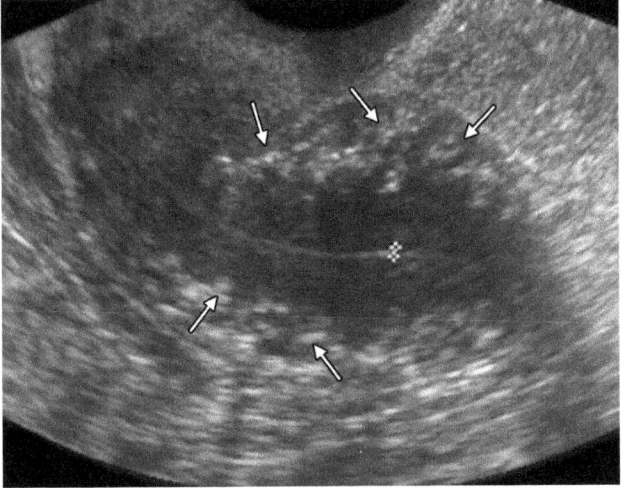

**Fig. 6.3:** Postmenopausal uterus with multiple foci of arcuate artery calcification.

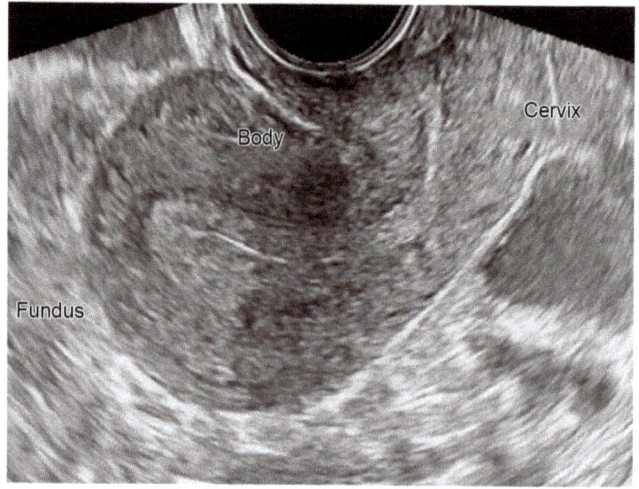

**Fig. 6.4:** The uterus has a fundus, body (corpus) and cervix.

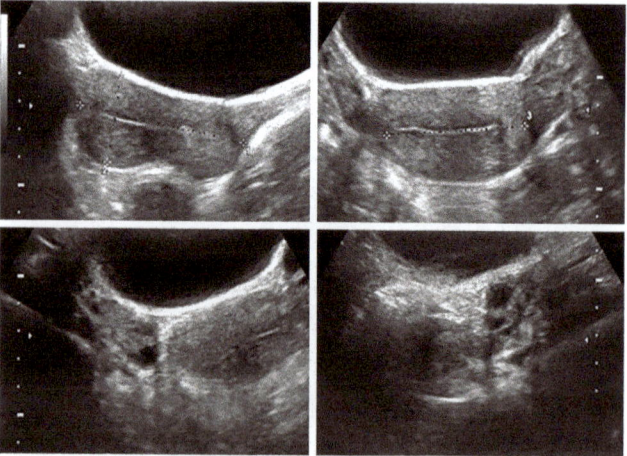

**Fig. 6.5:** Anteverted uterus seen on a transabdominal scan.

# Normal Female Pelvis

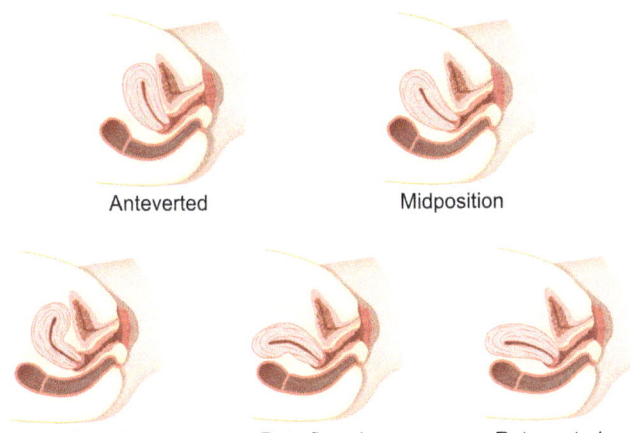

**Fig. 6.6:** Depending on the angle made by the cervix with the uterine corpus, the uterus is termed as anteverted or retroverted.

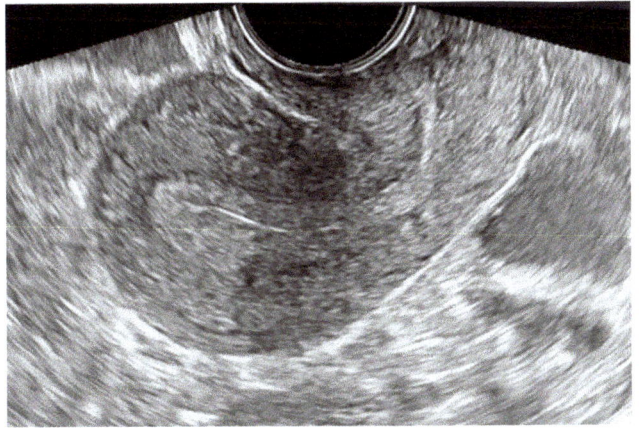

**Fig. 6.7:** Anteverted uterus seen on a transvaginal sonography (TVS)

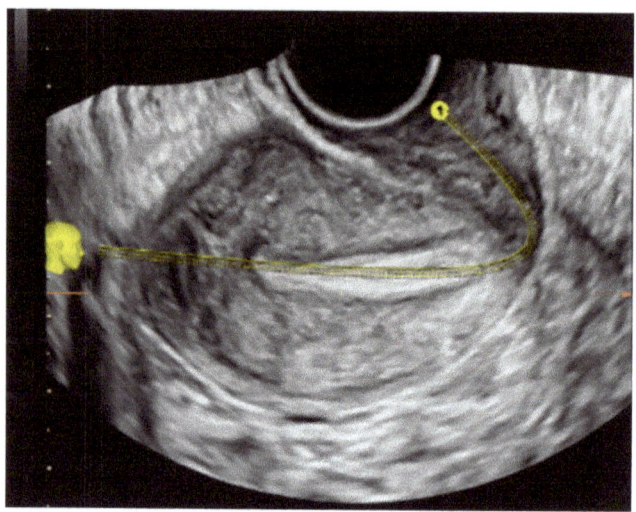

**Fig. 6.8:** Acutely anteverted uterus.

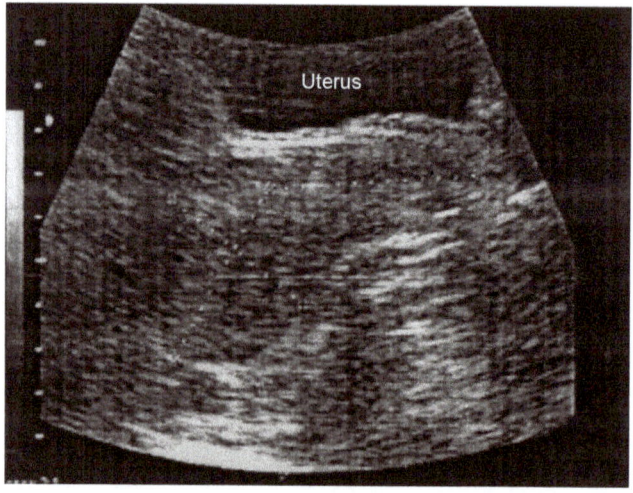

**Fig. 6.9:** Retroverted uterus as seen on TAS.

Normal Female Pelvis

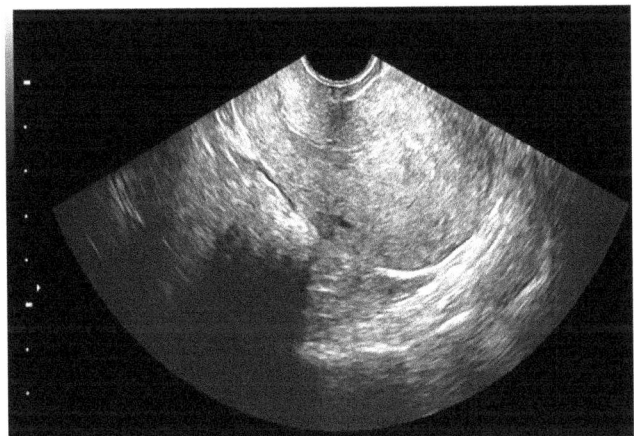

**Fig. 6.10:** A retroverted uterus which is going to be clearly seen with the probe being placed superior so that the tip of the probe points posteriorly.

cervix is homogeneous in echotexture with a hypoechoic central canal. Size of corpus relates to uterine cervix ratio which is 2:1. The uterine cervix has a length and diameter of 2.5 cm and is divided in vaginal and supravaginal part. Uterine arteries run along the sides of the cervix. Position of uterus is determined in relation to the vaginal and uterine longitudinal axis.

*Anteflexion*: Corpus of uterus bent forward in relation to cervical axis

*Anteversion*: Whole uterus bent forward in relation to vaginal axis

*Retroflexion*: Corpus of uterus bent backward in relation to cervical axis

*Retroversion*: Whole uterus bent backward in relation to vaginal axis.

## Layers

Uterine wall consists of 3 layers **(Figs. 6.11 to 6.20)**:
1. *Endometrium*: Inner most layer of uterus. It is further divided into two layers:
   a. *Basal layer (stratum basale)*: Deep endometrium layer which contains irregularly arranged glandular tubules. It does not shed during menstruation. It serves as a regenerative reservoir of cells for the functional layer.
   b. *Functional layer (stratum functionale)*: It is endometrium lies above the stratum basale, which sheds during menstruation.
2. *Myometrium*: It forms main bulk of the uterus. It comprises of interlacing smooth muscles fibers which

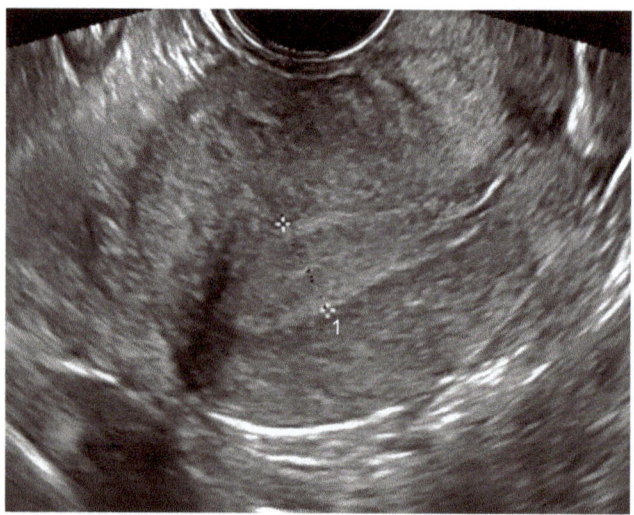

**Fig. 6.11:** Endometrial thickness, morphology and endometrial differentiation needs to be carefully checked.

Normal Female Pelvis

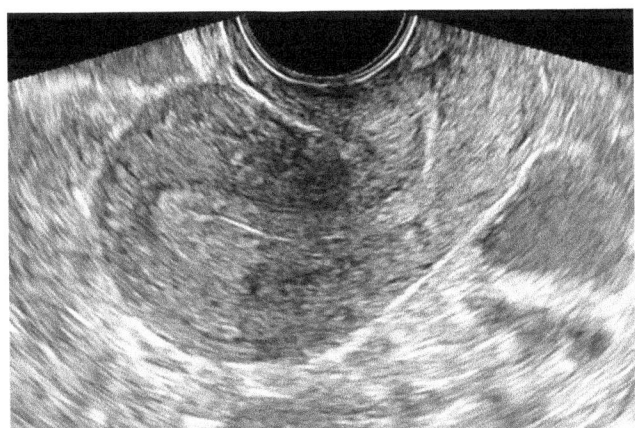

**Fig. 6.12:** The uterus has an endometrium which is visualized as a hyperechoic band in the center of the uterus and myometrium which should be homogeneous with smooth margins.

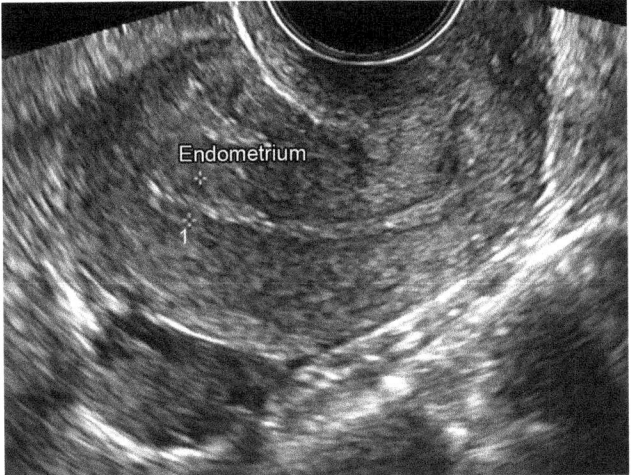

**Fig. 6.13:** Endometrium triple-layered as seen on TVS.

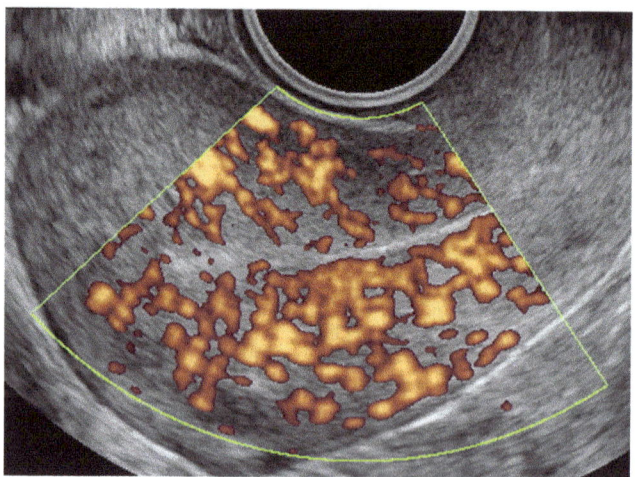

**Fig. 6.14:** Endometrium as seen on color flow imaging by TVS.

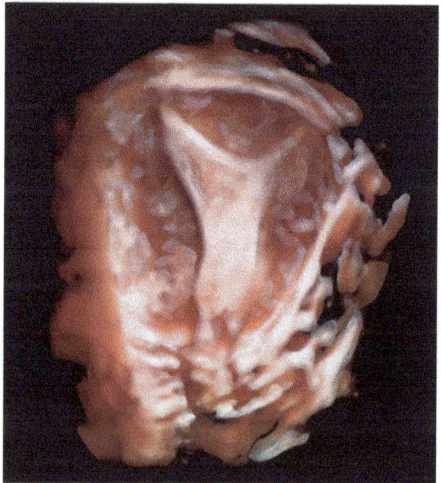

**Fig. 6.15:** Endometrium as seen on 3D.

Normal Female Pelvis

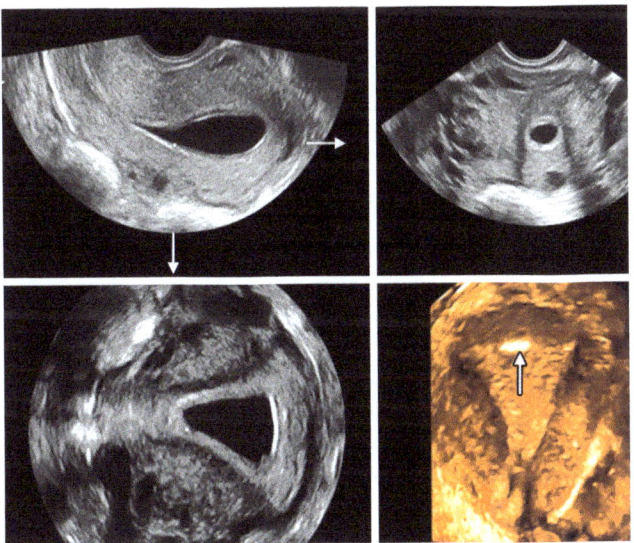

**Fig. 6.16:** Uterus as seen on multislice imaging.

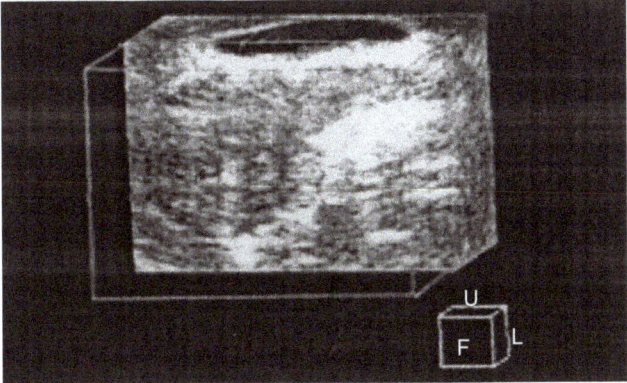

**Fig. 6.17:** Uterus as seen on sono CT.

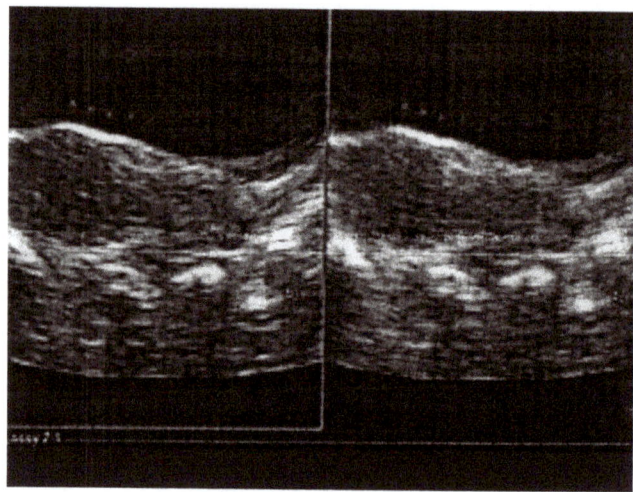

**Fig. 6.18:** Uterus as seen on sono MR.

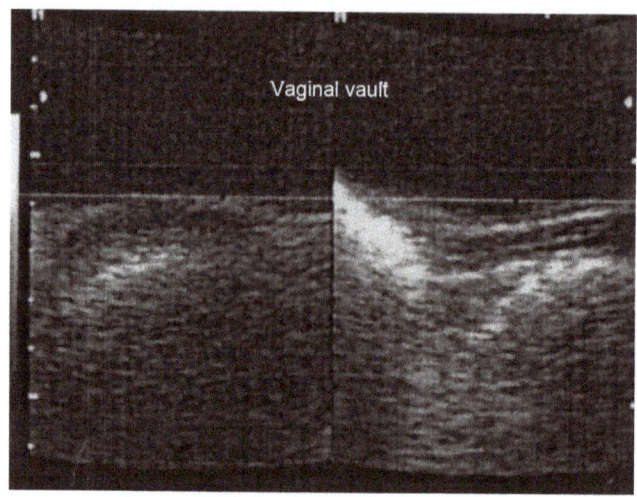

**Fig. 6.19:** Vaginal vault as seen on TAS.

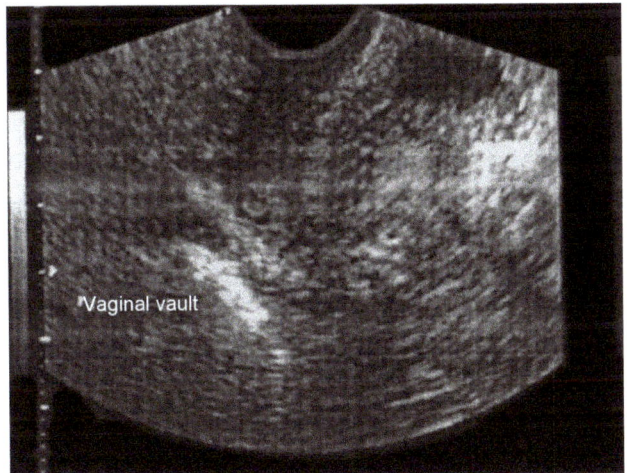

**Fig. 6.20:** Vaginal vault as seen on TVS.

intermingle with connective tissue, blood vessels, nerve and lymphatics. Smooth muscles fibers mainly longitudinal circular innermost, large intermediate layer arranged in criss-cross pattern and outer fibers are mostly arranged longitudinally.

3. *Perimetrium*: Outer layer of uterus, also a part of visceral peritoneum that spreads over bladder forms the vesicouterine pouch anteriorly, forms the rectouterine pouch (cul-de-sac) posteriorly, and forms broad ligament on each side of uterus laterally.

## FALLOPIAN TUBE

Fallopian tube also called oviduct or uterine tube derived from Müllerian ducts arise from the cornual end of uterus. They serve as conveyer for ovary and the sperm for fertilization. 9–11 cm long, spread along the upper margins of broad ligament, endoperitoneal cavity close to the ovary. Opening is called abdominal opening, it has a finger-like projection called fimbriae which plays an important role in fertility as they pickup the oocyte at time of ovulation.

It has four parts.
1. *Interstitial/intramural part:* 1 cm long, 1 mm in diameter, lies embedded in the uterine wall.
2. *Isthmic part*: Medial part of tube between interstitial and ampullary. Narrower part 1–2 mm in diameter.
3. Ampulla lies between isthmic and infundibulum thin wall, tortous, 5 cm long, comprises 2/3rd of tubal length. Site of fertilization.
4. *Infundibulum*: Peritoneal opening of fallopian tube 2 cm large, its ends has figure-like projections called fimbriae.

Arterial supply terminal branches of uterine and ovarian arteries.

*Venous Drainage:* Parallel to the arterial supply.

Fallopian tube composed of three layers. *Outer* serosal layer consists of peritoneum and underlying layers of connective tissue.

*Middle* muscular layer consists of outer longitudinal fibers and inner circular ones.

*Inner* mucus layer, lined with columnar epithelium which contains cilia which with the help of peristaltic action help in ovum and sperm transport.

# OVARIES (FIGS. 6.21 TO 6.37)

These are positioned on each side of the cervix in the ovarian fossa adjacent to the lateral wall and is delineated with the

## Normal Female Pelvis

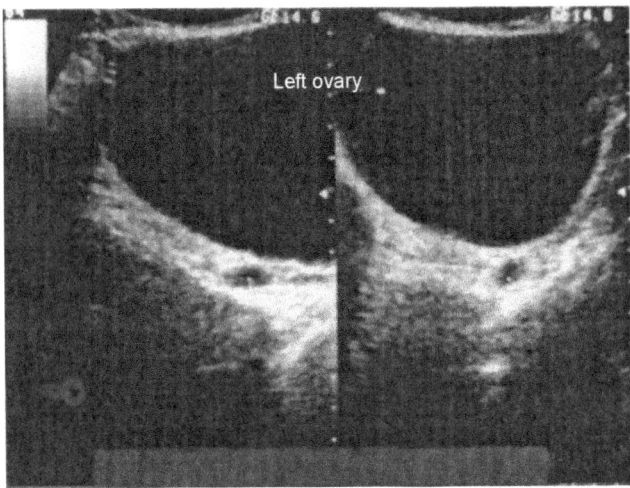

**Fig. 6.21:** Ovaries in a prepubertal female.

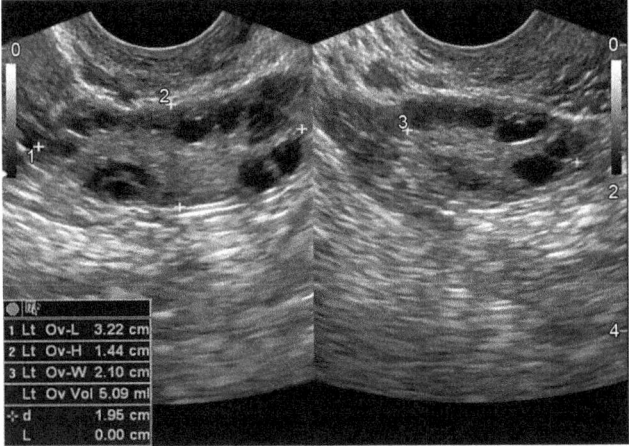

**Fig. 6.22:** Ovaries in a postpubertal female which are ovoid in shape and generally measure 30 × 20 × 20 mm.

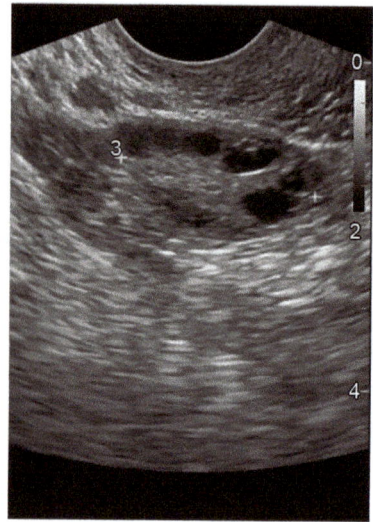

**Fig. 6.23:** Normal ovary as seen on TVS.

ureter and the internal iliac vessels. The ovary is attached to the posterior layer of broad ligament by meso-ovarium, to the lateral pelvic wall by infundibulopelvic ligament and to the uterus by the ovarian ligament.

## Size

Ovaries in girls younger than 2 years of age are typically less than 1 mL in volume, although in neonates they can be slightly larger. The ovaries increase in size in prepubertal girls with follicles up to 1 cm in size. After menarche, the ovaries are ovoid in shape and generally measure 30 × 20 × 10 mm. Paired sex gonads which are concerned with germ cell maturation, storage and its release and steroidogenesis.

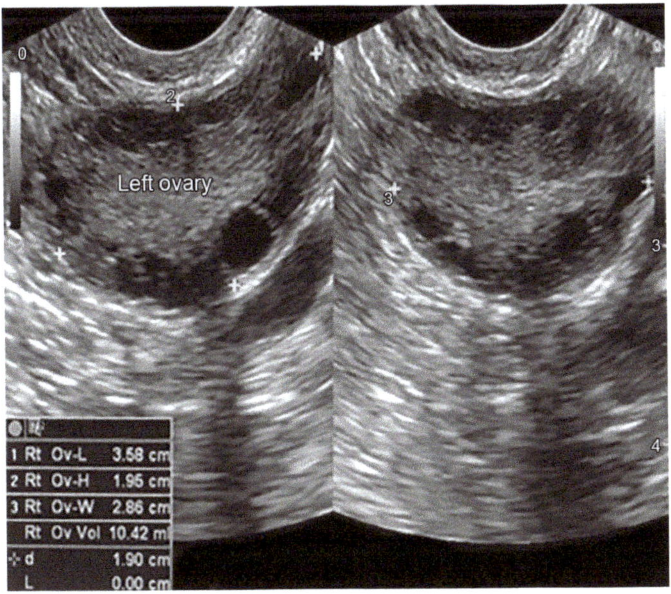

## Normal Female Pelvis

**Fig. 6.24:** In the proliferative phase of the menstrual cycle, multiple small follicles are visualized, usually 10 mm in diameter or less. Small 07 mm follicle seen on the 8th day of the cycle.

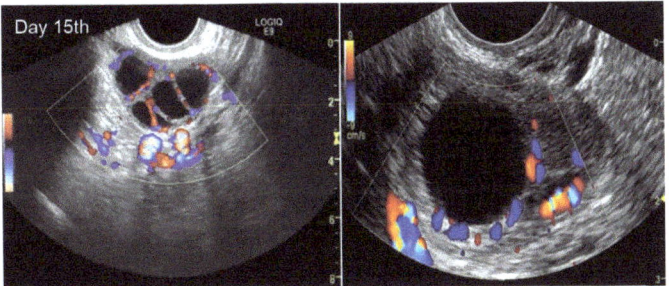

**Fig. 6.25:** Ovary with maturing follicle as seen on TVS.

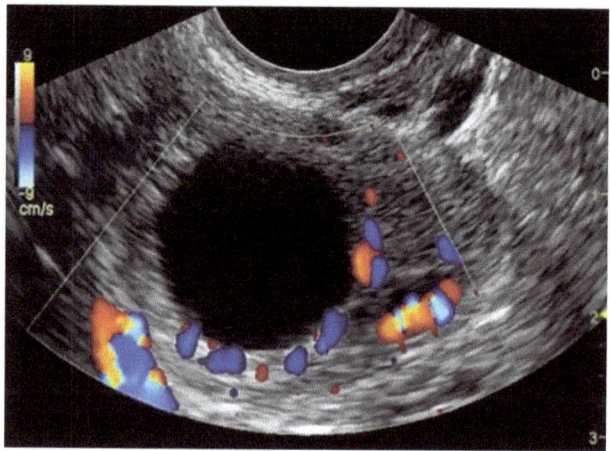

**Fig. 6.26:** 17 mm maturing follicle as seen on TVS.

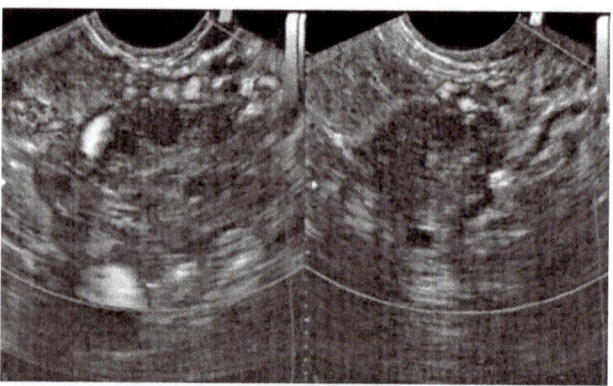

**Fig. 6.27:** Ovary seen medial to the iliac vessel.

It measures 3 cm × 2 cm × 1 cm, length, breath and thickness.

*Arterial supply* from ovarian artery branch of abdominal aorta.

Normal Female Pelvis

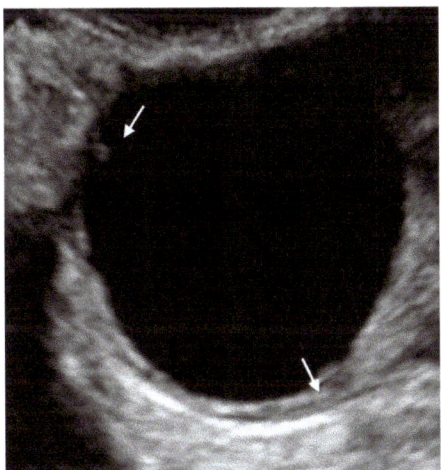

**Fig. 6.28:** The follicle increases in size and a 16 mm maturing follicle is seen on the 11th day of the cycle.

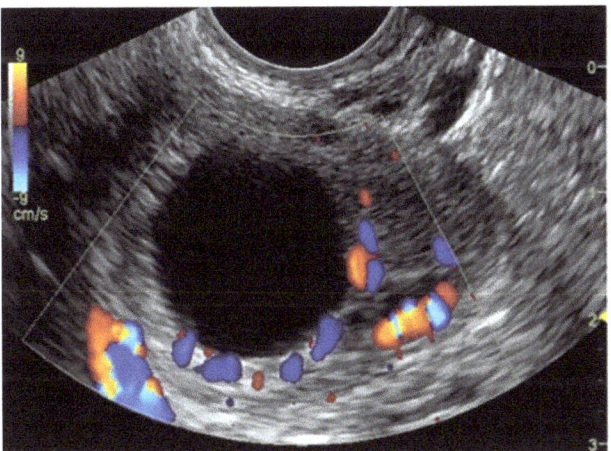

**Fig. 6.29:** A dominant follicle is seen in the midcycle, which measures 19 mm in diameter.

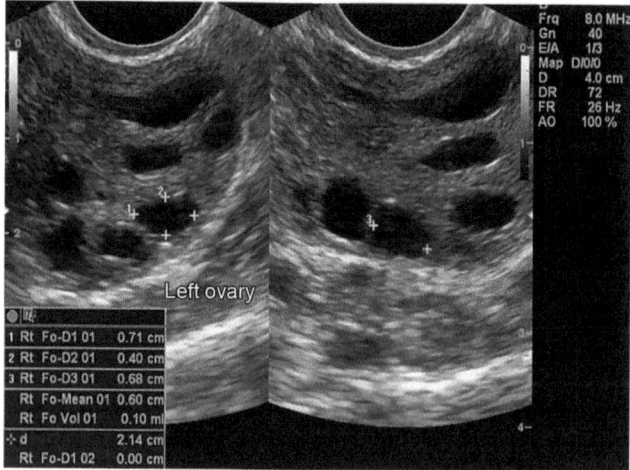

**Fig. 6.30:** Ovary with multiple small follicles seen after stimulation.

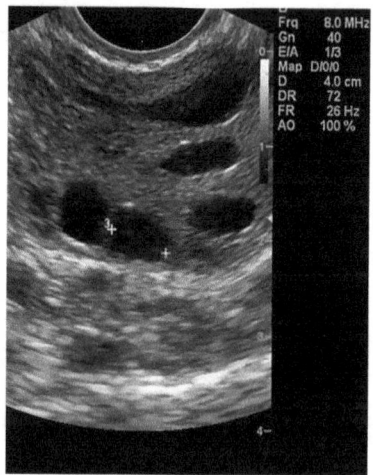

**Fig. 6.31:** In patients with stimulation multiple follicles are seen.

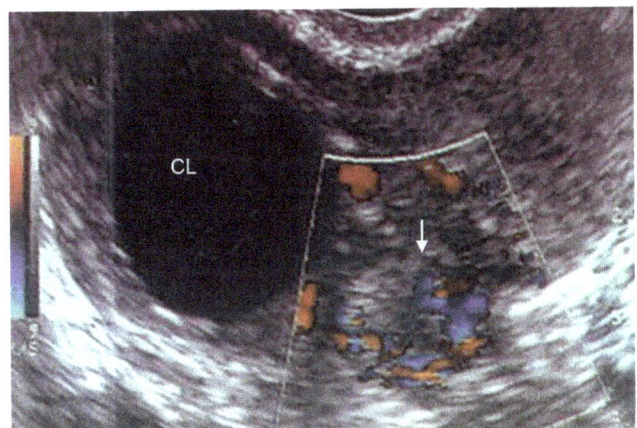

**Fig. 6.32:** After ovulation, the corpus luteum (CL) cyst is seen as a hypoechoic area within the ovary.

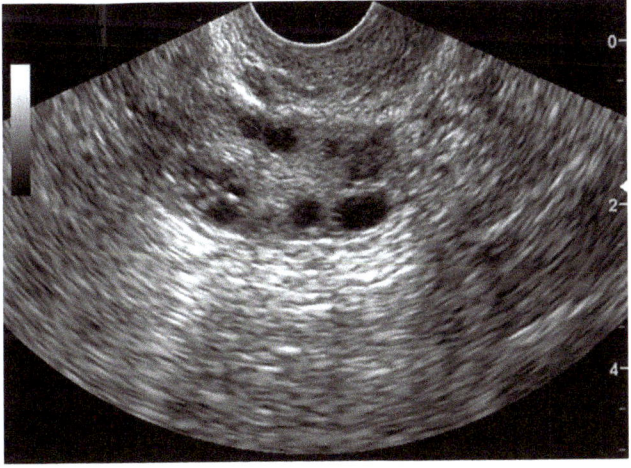

**Fig. 6.33:** Ovary in a postmenopausal female.

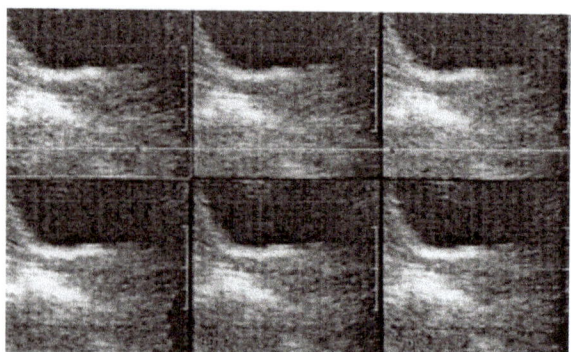

**Fig. 6.34:** Ovary as seen on multislice imaging.

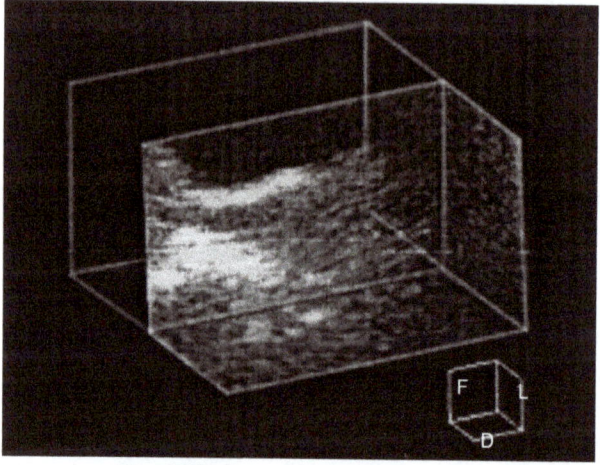

**Fig. 6.35:** Ovary as seen on sono CT.

*Venous drainage* through pampiniform plexus, to form the ovarian veins which drain into inferior vena cava on the right side and left renal vein on the left side.

*Nerve supply:* Sympathetic supply comes down along the ovarian artery from $T_{10}$ segment.

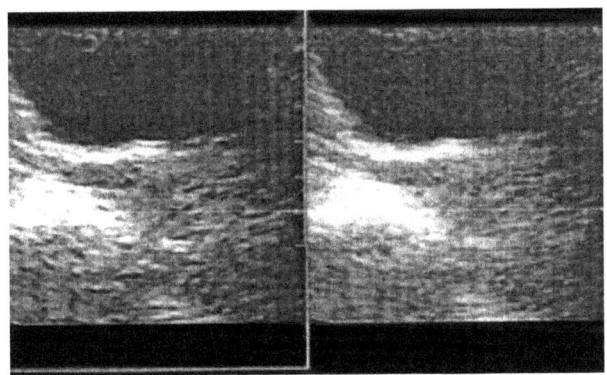

**Fig. 6.36:** Ovary as seen on sono MR.

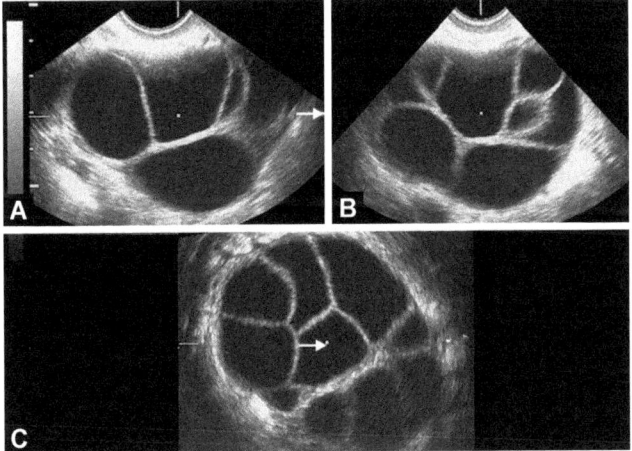

**Figs. 6.37A to C:** 3D of ovarian volume in a hyperstimulated ovary.

## Folliculogenesis

Folliculogenesis is a continuous process, which starts in embryonic period and ends with the disappearance of the last functional follicle in the period of menopause.

It refers to all phases that a primordial germ cell has to pass to become a mature healthy oocyte for fertilization with the sperm.

The development of primordial to full grown secondary follicles requires 290 days or about 10 regular menstrual cycles.

Healthy antral follicles measuring 2–5 mm that are present during the late luteal phase of preceding cycle, constitutes the population from which the follicle destined to ovulate in the subsequent cycle. These follicles called recruited follicles. Number varies 3–11 per ovary in women aged 24–35 years. Then these recruited follicles of preceding cycle, follicle selection occurs which presumed to occur during the first five days of next cycle when the leading follicular diameter is 5–10 mm.

Selected follicles become dominant between 5 and 7 days of cycle when the follicles diameter is approx 10 mm.

After attaining dominance it grows at a rate of 2–3 mm/day until it reaches a near diameter ranging from 17 to 27 mm just prior to ovulation.

Under the influence of midcycle LH large ovulation occurs which consists of rapid follicular enlargement followed by perfusion of follicle from surface of ovarian cortex. Finally follicles ruptures and oocyte-cumulus complex extrude which is picked by fimbriae of fallopian tube.

After ovulation, granular cell becomes luteinized and gives rise to corpus luteum. It is highly vascularized endocrine gland, which is a source of progesterone in secretory phase of cycle to support the endometrium. If pregnancy does not occur, corpus luteum regress via a process called autolysis. If pregnancy occurs hCG secreted by trophoblast maintain the viability of corpus luteum to produce progesterone until the cutco placental shift occurs.

## POUCH OF DOUGLAS (FIG. 6.38)

A small amount of fluid is present in the cul-de-sac of asymptomatic women throughout the menstrual cycle. This increases at the time of ovulation. Fluid in cul-de-sac act as a contrast medium to visualize to normal fallopian tube. Blood may be present in the pelvis in case of rupture of corpus rectum, rupture of ectopic pregnancy.

Remember whenever you see any pathology you are supposed to be mentioning the size, echo pattern, if possible mobility, if you have a color Doppler the vascularity and the organ of origin of the lesion. Do not tend to give a histopathological diagnosis because there are so many overlaps. Ultrasound can make anatomical diagnosis and not cytological or histopathological diagnosis.

## DOPPLER EVALUATION OF PELVIC VISCERA

- Can evaluate pelvic vascular anatomy
- Iliac, uterine and ovarian flows

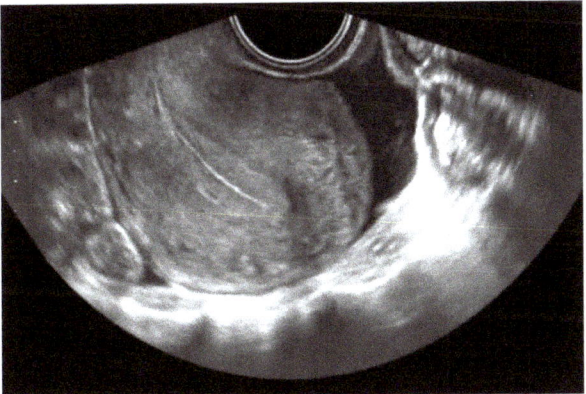

**Fig. 6.38:** A small amount of fluid is present in the cul-de-sac of asymptomatic women throughout the menstrual cycle.

- Can be identified and pulsed Doppler can analyze the velocity and waveform
- Important to know woman's menstrual dates to interpret the wave
- The three arteries have a different and characteristic wave pattern
- Color, pulsed, angio, 3D power, CVI all have a definite place in pelvic evaluation
- Normal and abnormal vasculature
- Benign and malignant masses
- Trophoblastic flow and ectopic pregnancy
- Vasculature of fibroids and ovarian cysts, torsion, inflammation of masses.

## 3D EVALUATION OF PELVIC VISCERA

- Evaluation of uterine cavity with simultaneous presentation of all three planes
- Noninvasive and accurate assessment of congenital uterine anomalies
- Precise ovarian volume measurements
- Accurately detect the cumulus oophorus
- 3D power Doppler for distinguishing normal from pathological angiogenesis
- 3D volume and 3D power Doppler visualize more precisely pathological processes in the fallopian tubes.
    - Exact volume measurement of endometrial hyperplasia
    - Virtual hysteroscopy (3D/4D), using slicing technique
    - Exact localization and measurement of ovarian and endometrial tumor
    - Tumor monitoring after treatment.
    - Contrast media to check tumor visualization and blood supply and for follow-up after (4D).

# CHAPTER 7

# Uterine Disorders

Evaluation of the uterus comprises of checking for **(Figs. 7.1 to 7.3)**:
- Size
- Shape
- Position
- Surface
- Mobility
- Tenderness

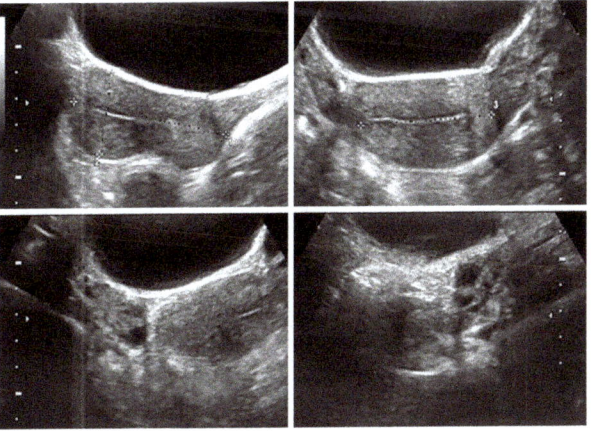

**Fig. 7.1:** Normal uterus and cervix as seen on a transabdominal sonography (TAS).

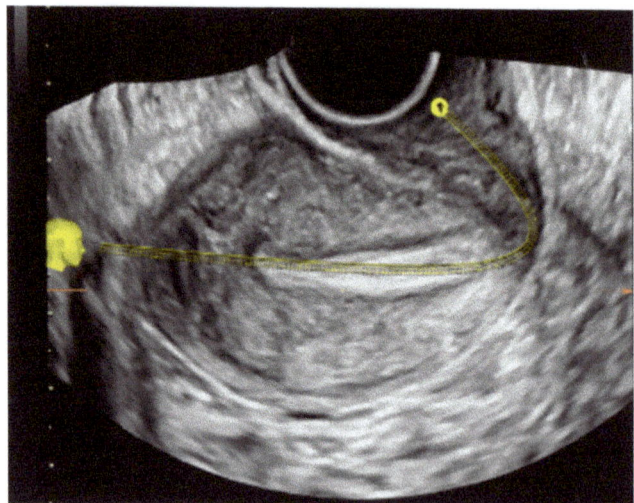

**Fig. 7.2:** Acutely anteverted uterus as seen on a transvaginal sonography (TVS).

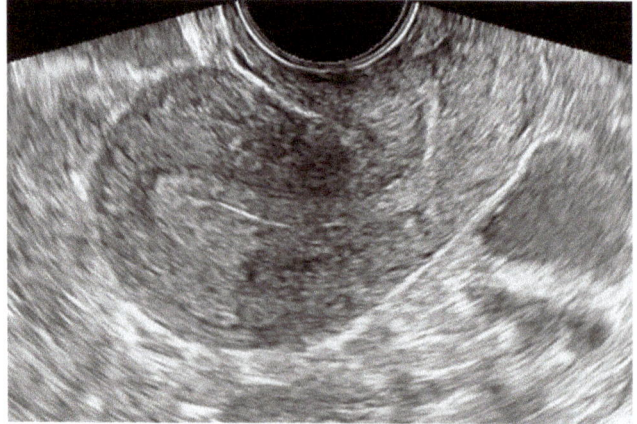

**Fig. 7.3:** Uterus as seen on a TVS.

Uterine Disorders

The areas one needs to check in the uterus are:
- Uterine musculature
- Uterine cavity
- Endometrium
- Color flows
- Endometrial scoring (USSR)

## MYOMETRIUM

In the myometrium one has to check for:
- Fibroids
- Adenomyosis
- Myometritis
- Calcifications
- Size of uterus
- Shape
- Position
- Mobility
- Probe tenderness.

## Fibroids (Figs. 7.4 to 7.31)

Most common tumors of reproductive age group, benign tumors of smooth muscles cells of uterus, estrogen dependent, size increases in pregnancy and decreases after menopause.
- Salient features to be evaluated in fibroids are:
  - Number of fibroids
  - Size of fibroids
  - Position of fibroids
  - Color flow in fibroids
  - Degenerative changes.
- Fibroids are described by their location. They can be submucosal (displacing/distorting the endometrium),

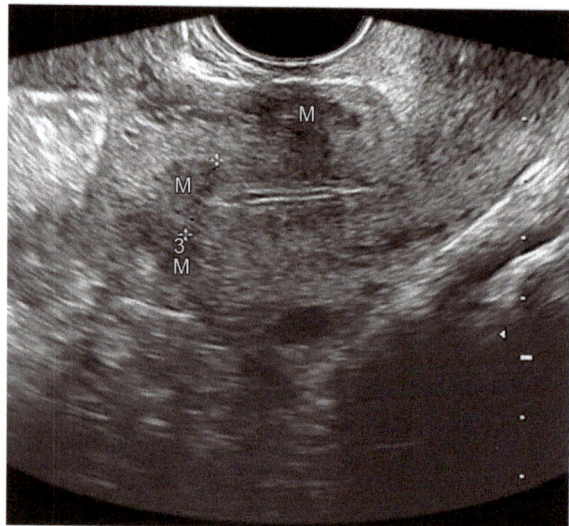

**Fig. 7.4:** Multiple submucosal and intramural fibroids.

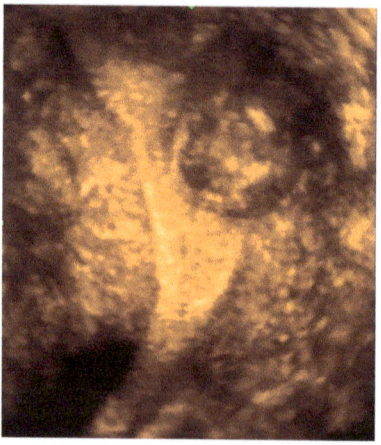

**Fig. 7.5:** 3D image—large left lateral wall fibroid with indentation on the endometrial cavity—also seen the cornual extension.

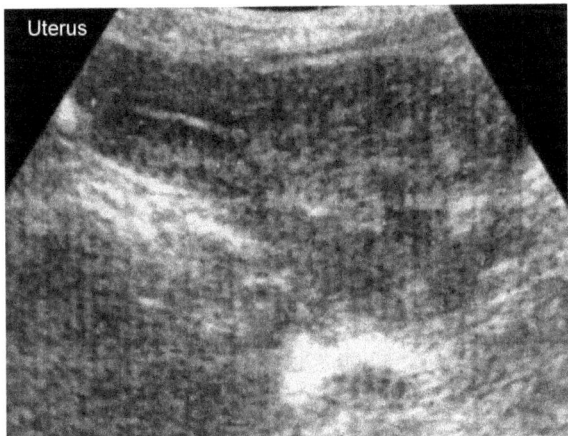

**Fig. 7.6:** Pedunculated fibroid seen in the uterine corpus and through the cervical canal.

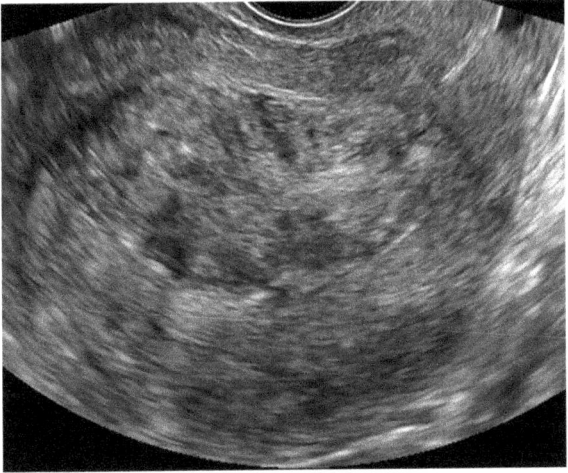

**Fig. 7.7:** Hyaline degeneration (irregular anechoic areas in the fibroid with no distal acoustic enhancement) in a posterior wall panmural fibroid.

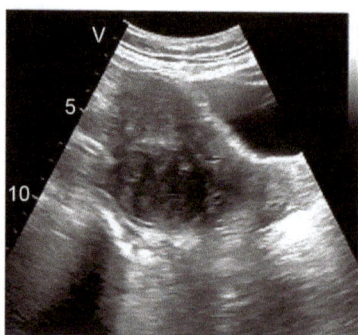

**Fig. 7.8:** Cystic degeneration (irregular anechoic areas in the fibroid with distal acoustic enhancement) in a fundal panmural fibroid.

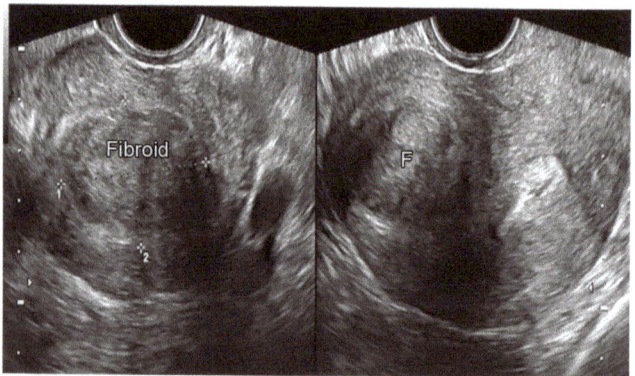

**Fig. 7.9:** Relationship of the endometrium with the panmural fibroid.

intramural (within the wall of the uterus and not distorting either the endometrial cavity or the uterine contour), subserosal (seen distorting the uterine contour), panmural (through and through from the outer surface till the endometrial cavity) or pedunculated, cervical fibroid and intraligamentary.

# Uterine Disorders

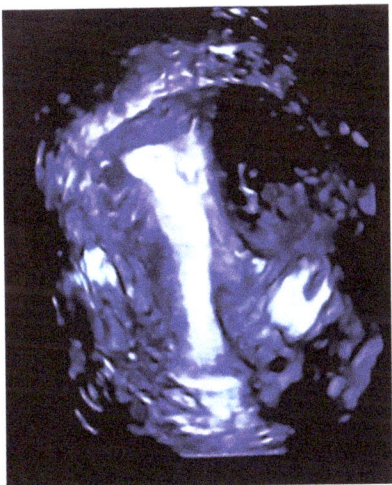

**Fig. 7.10:** Same fibroid seen on 3D.

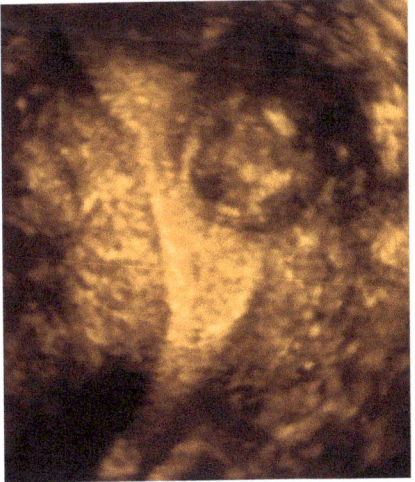

**Fig. 7.11:** One can appreciate the degeneration on 3D.

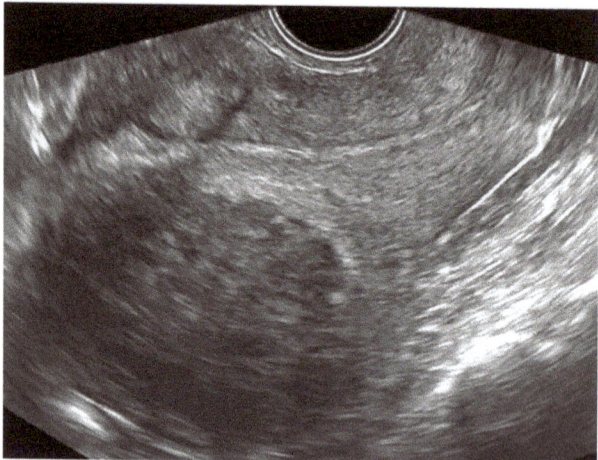

**Fig. 7.12:** Large posterior wall panmural fibroid.

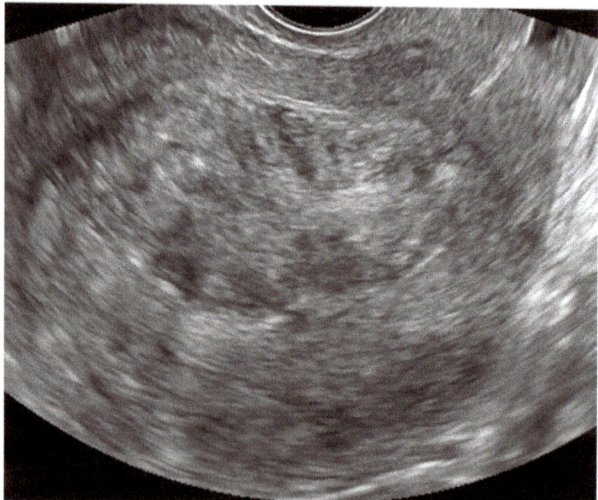

**Fig. 7.13:** Anterior wall—near complete panmural fibroid—more so intramural.

Uterine Disorders

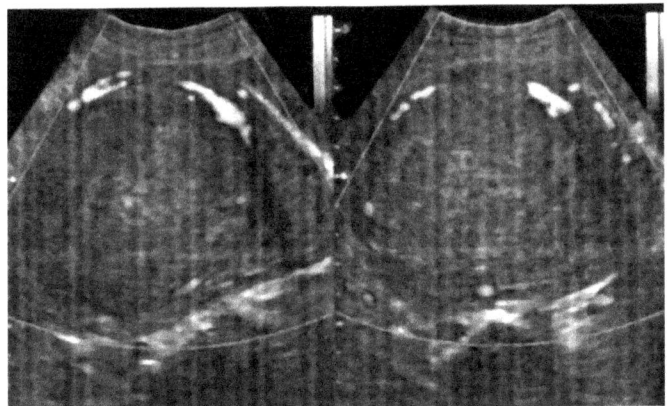

**Fig. 7.14:** Fundal panmural fibroid.

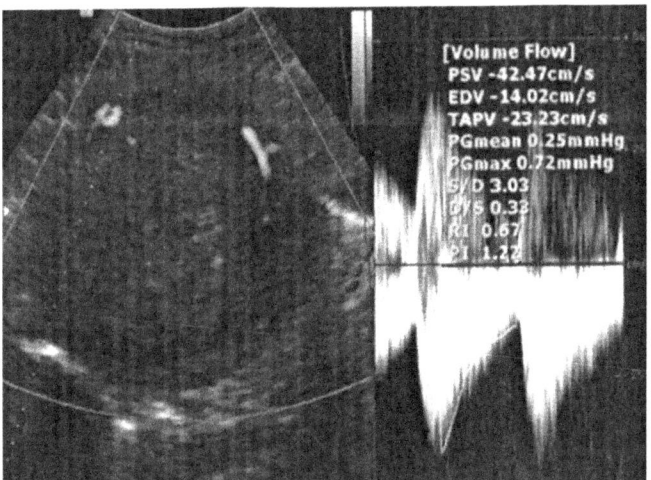

**Fig. 7.15:** Fundal panmural fibroid with peripheral vessels showing high impedance flow as seen on color flow mapping and duplex Doppler.

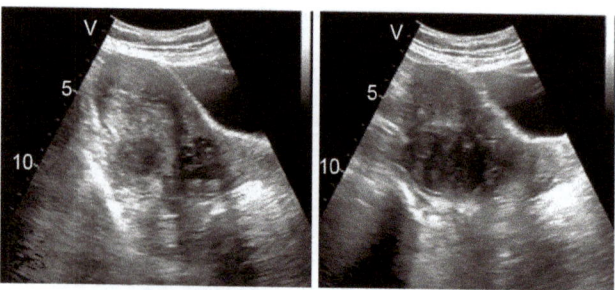

**Fig. 7.16:** Posterior wall subserous fibroid (TAS).

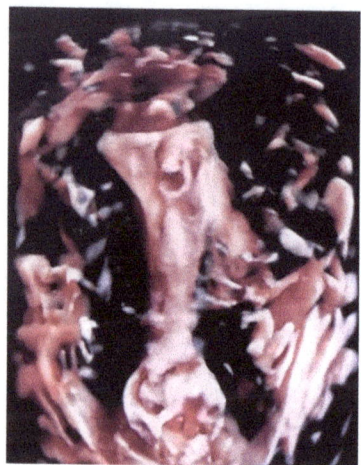

**Fig. 7.17:** Left cornual fibroid and submucosal fibroid seen on rendered 3D HD live image.

## Ultrasound Features of Fibroids

- Uterine enlargement
- Distortion of uterine contour
- Depending on the amount of connective tissue and smooth muscles, they may be isoechoic, hypoechoic, hyperechoic

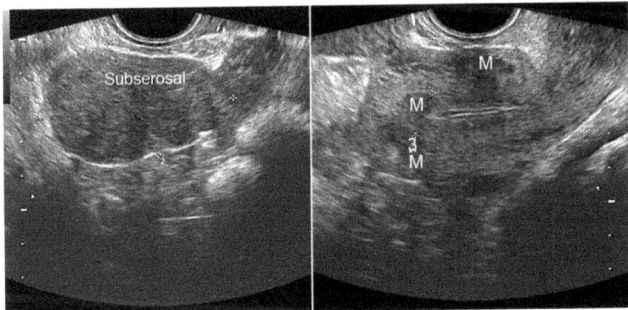

**Fig. 7.18:** Anterior and posterior wall subserous fibroids.

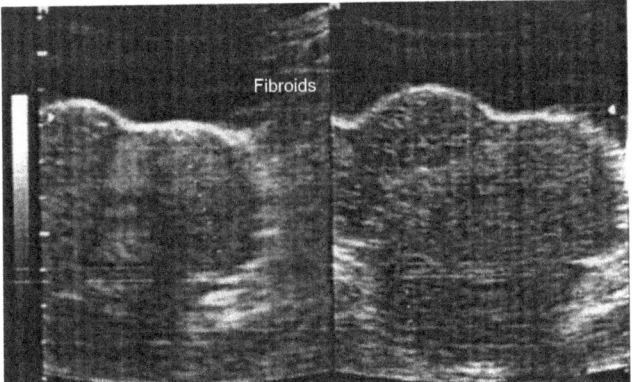

**Fig. 7.19:** Left wall and right wall subserous fibroids seen.

- On color Doppler they show peripheral vascularization suggestive of uterine origin with RI $0.54 \pm 0.08$
- In case of necrosis, inflammation and degenerative changes, they may show central vascularization with low RI values.
- Fibroids assessed on 2D, but their exact location difficult to determine due to shadowing and artifacts 3D overcomes these difficulties, by allowing visualization in

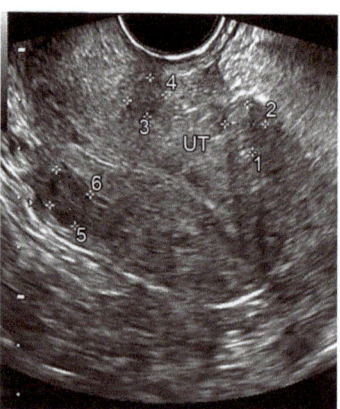

**Fig. 7.20:** Interstitial and subserous fibroids.

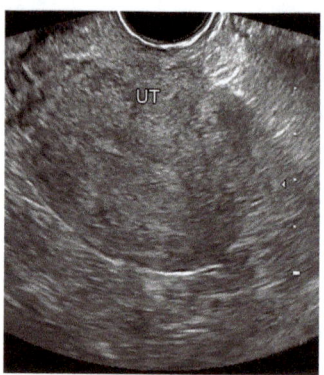

**Fig. 7.21:** Multiple interstitial fibroids seen in the uterus myometrium.

coronal plane, 3D demonstrates exact location of fibroids and the plan of management.

### *Leiomyosarcoma*

Rare tumors, 3–7.4% of malignant tumors of genital tract.

## Uterine Disorders

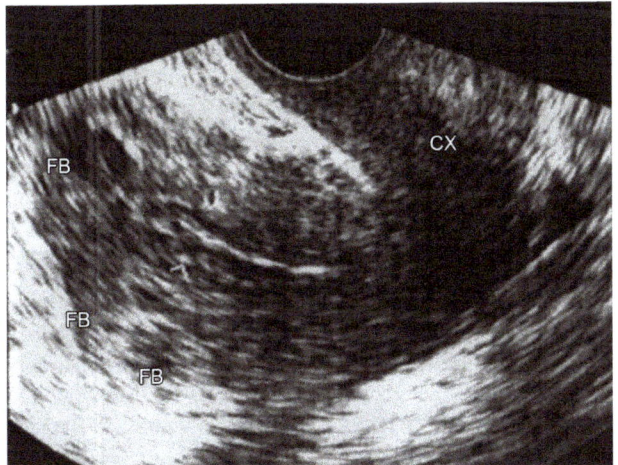

**Fig. 7.22:** Multiple seedling fibroids (FB) which are subserous along the anterior and posterior uterine wall.

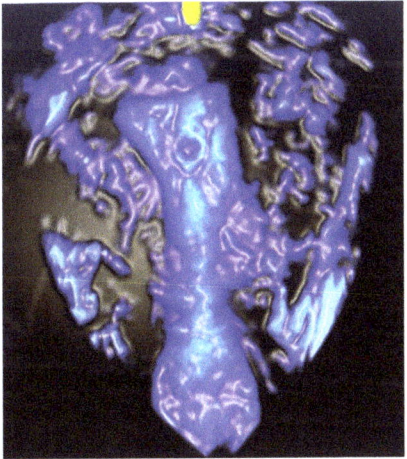

**Fig. 7.23:** 3D image of submucosal fibroid and intramural fibroid indenting the cavity.

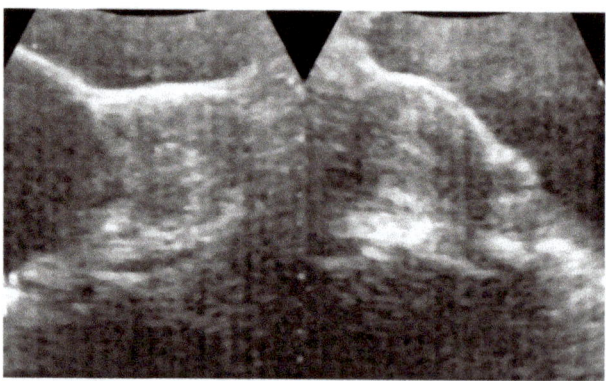

**Fig. 7.24:** Two right wall interstitial fibroids (within the wall of the uterus and not distorting either the endometrial cavity or the uterine contour).

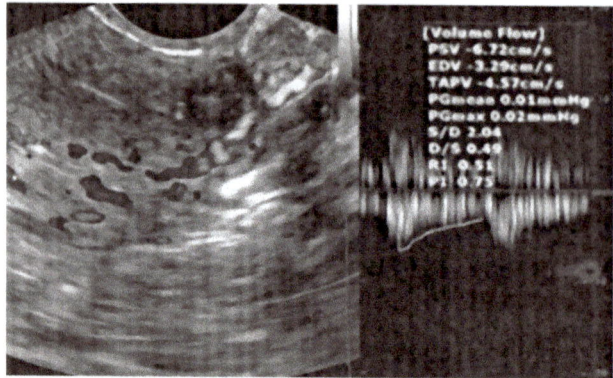

**Fig. 7.25:** Left wall interstitial fibroid which is mildly vascular on color floor imaging.

## USG Features

Solid or solid-cystic structure altering echogenicity of the myometrium and neovascularization optional of the tumor.

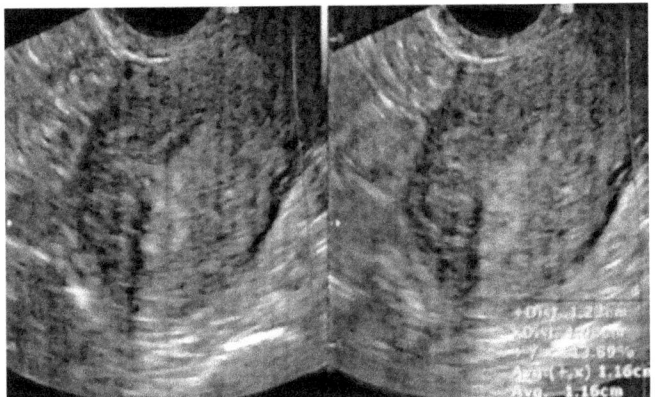

**Fig. 7.26:** Anterior wall submucous fibroid seen indenting the endometrium.

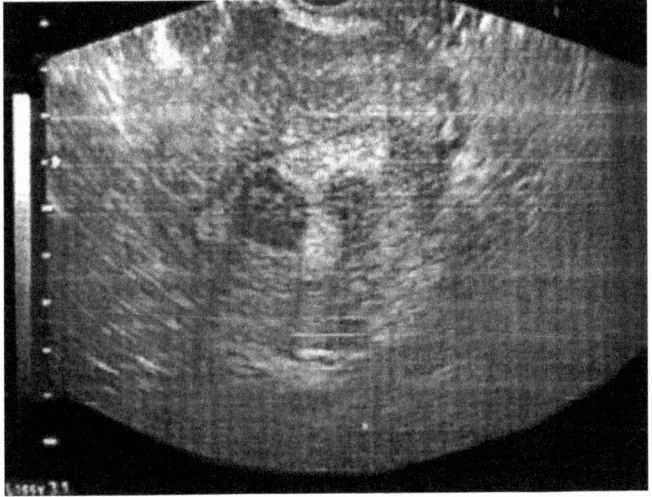

**Fig. 7.27:** Fibroid polyps (hypoechoic) as opposed to endometrial polyps (hyperechoic) seen in the uterine cavity.

# 110  Ultrasound in Gynecology

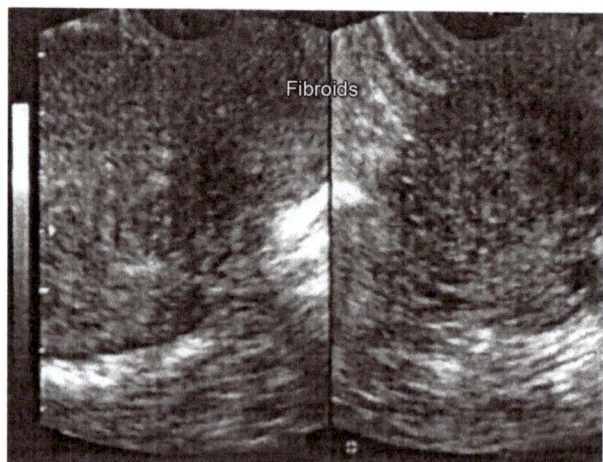

**Fig. 7.28:** Submucous fibroid in the uterine corpus within the uterine cavity.

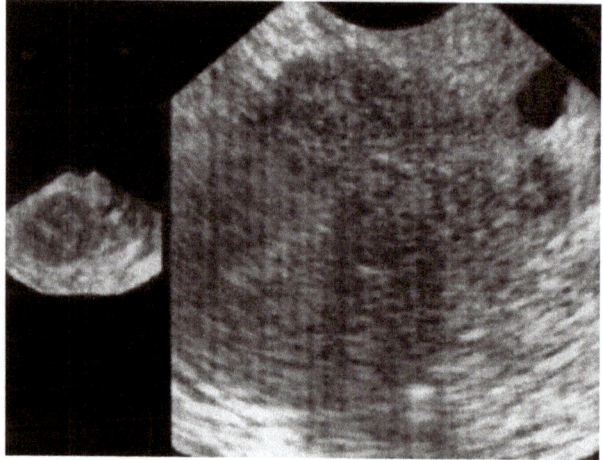

**Fig. 7.29:** Posterior wall submucous fibroid (displacing/distorting the endometrium).

Uterine Disorders

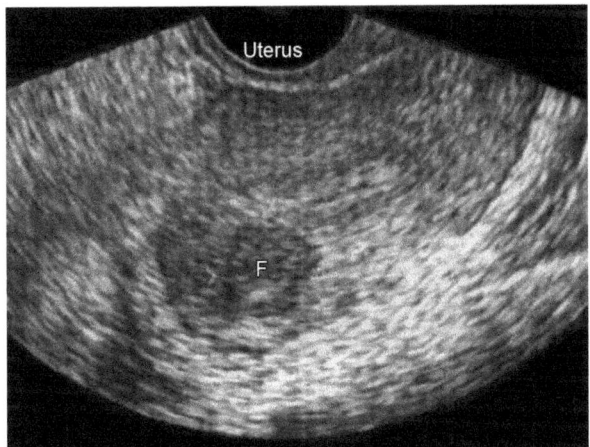

**Fig. 7.30:** Posterior wall submucous fibroid in the subfundal area (14 × 13 mm across) displacing the endometrium.

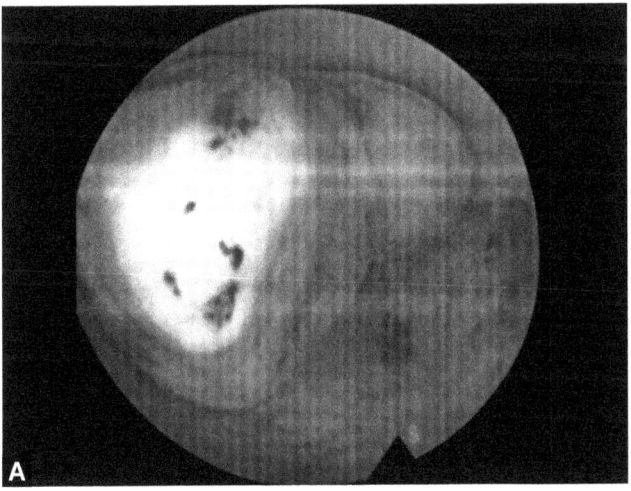

**Fig. 7.31A**

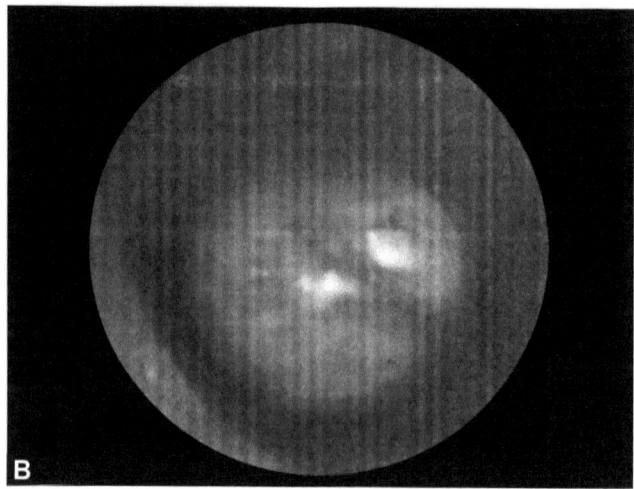

**Figs. 7.31A and B:** Submucous fibroids as seen through a hysteroscope.

On CD, high blood flow velocity and low resistance to blood flow within irregular, randomly dispersed thin vessels are seen.

RI = 0.37 ± 0.03

## Symptoms

### Complications of Fibroid

Fibroids can undergo atrophic, hyaline (irregular anechoic areas in the fibroid with no distal acoustic enhancement), cystic (irregular anechoic areas in the fibroid with distal acoustic enhancement), myxomatous, lipomatous, calcific (high level echoes within the fibroid with distal acoustic shadowing) and carneous degeneration and infarction, infection, torsion and malignant change.

## Adenomyosis (Figs. 7.32 to 7.35)

Also called uterine endometriosis. It is a condition in which endometrial tissue invades the myometrium. Affects 20% women, mainly multiparous.

USG features:
- Disturbed echogenicity of middle myometrial layer.

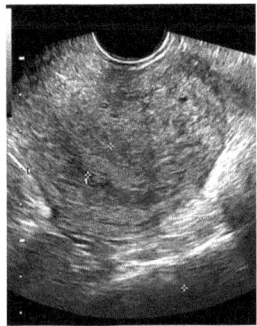

**Fig. 7.32:** Adenomyotic uterus with a diffuse speckled appearance of the myometrium.

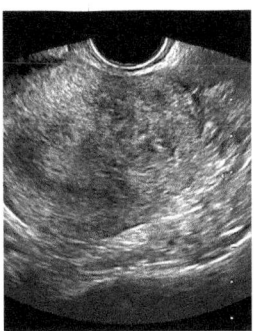

**Fig. 7.33:** An enlarged, globular and bosselated adenomyotic uterus.

- Multiple small cysts in myometrium called Swiss cheese appearance or salt and pepper appearance due to areas of hemorrhage and clots within the myometrium.

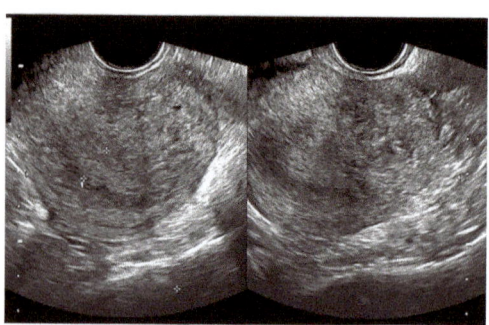

**Fig. 7.34:** Characteristic speckling of the myometrium seen with a thicker posterior myometrium than anterior myometrium.

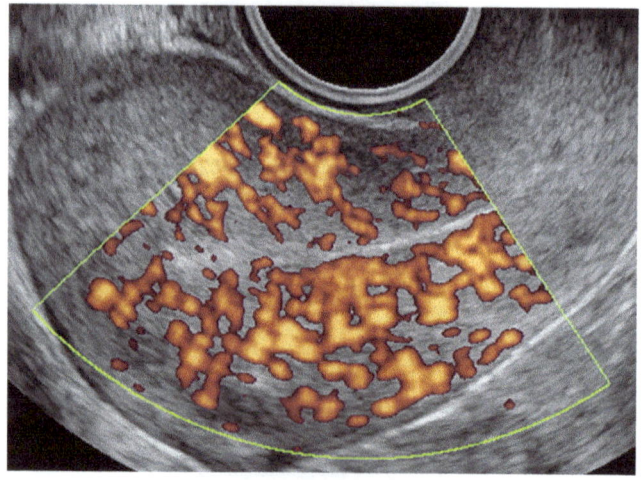

**Fig. 7.35**

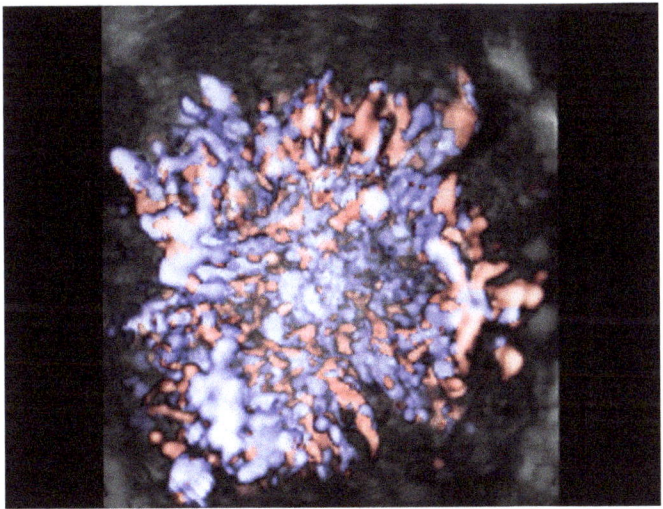

**Fig. 7.35:** Power Doppler and 3D rendered Doppler image.

- Hypoechoic myometrium.
- On CD study shows increased vascularity within the myometrium. RI = 0.56 ± 0.12
- Loss of endometrial myometrial junction.
- Images show "venetian blind" shadow of diffuse adenomyosis.
- 3D ultrasound particularly useful for assessing two functional zone or coronal plane on 3D JZ layer ≥ 4 mm and JZ infiltration and distortion of JZ made out clearly which is impossible to delineate on 2D ultrasound.

## Obstruction (Figs. 7.36 to 7.40)

Patients with hydrocolpos (fluid in the vagina) and hydrometrocolpos (fluid in the vagina and uterus) usually are seen soon after birth or at puberty when secretions cause

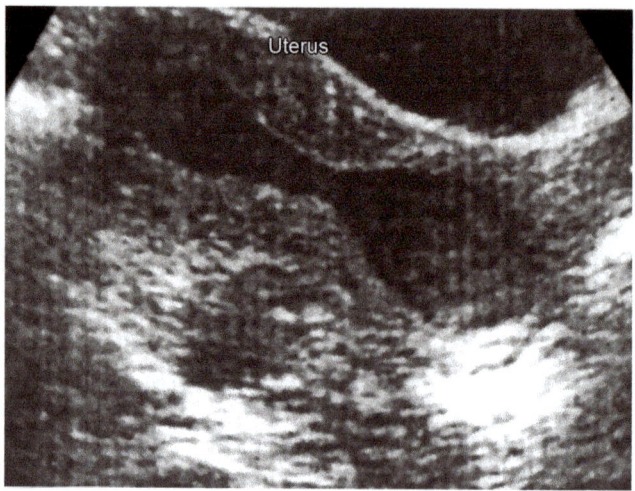

**Fig. 7.36:** Hydrometrocolpos (fluid in the vagina and uterus) seen at puberty when secretions cause obstruction because of an intact hymen or vaginal atresia.

obstruction because of an intact hymen or vaginal atresia. Hematometra is also seen in patients with cervical cancer or cervical stenosis.

## Uterine Calcifications (Figs. 7.41 and 7.42)

The most common cause of dense echoes in the uterus are calcifications resulting from fibroids. Less common cause of calcification within the uterus are that of the arcuate artery calcification, most commonly seen in postmenopausal women and woman with hypertension.

**Myometritis:** Inflammation of myometrium, seen in patient of pelvic inflammatory disease (PID) and postpartum patients.

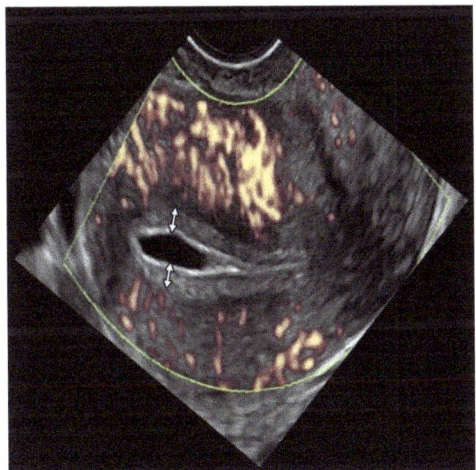

**Fig. 7.37:** Exclude the fluid collection to measure the endometrial thickness.

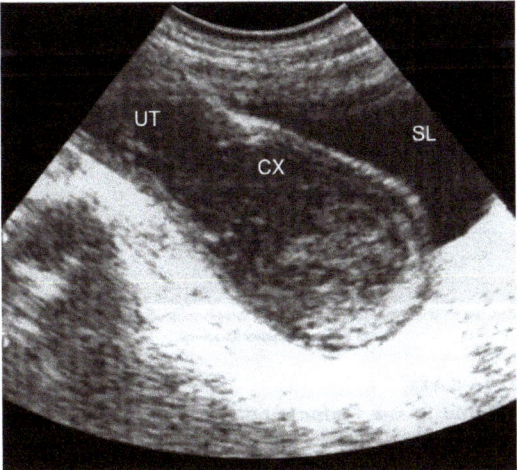

**Fig. 7.38:** Fluid collection seen in the cervix and uterus.

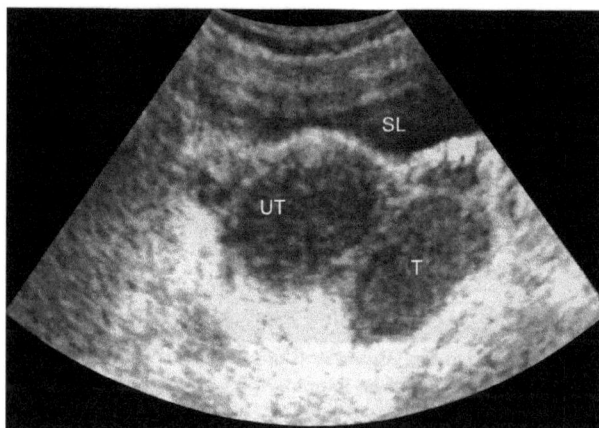

**Fig. 7.39:** Same patient showing a fluid collection in the tubes as well (hematosalpinx).

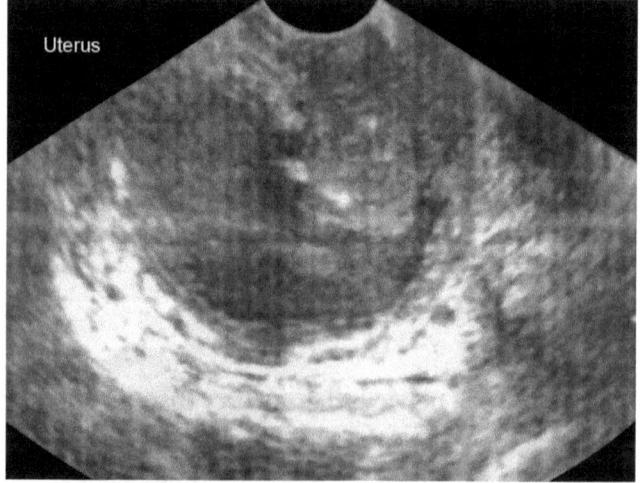

**Fig. 7.40:** Hematometra seen in patients with cervical cancer. Note the atrophic myometrium with calcific foci.

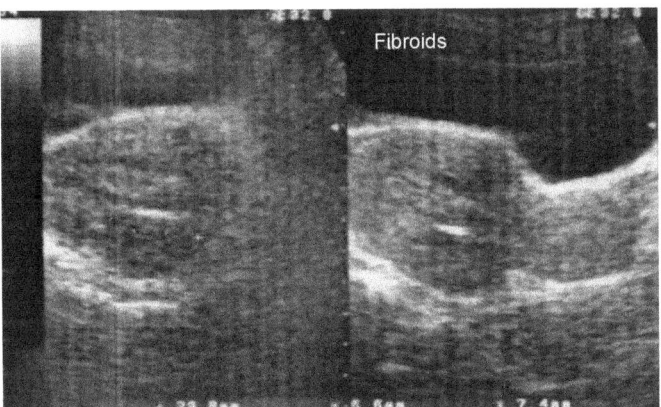

**Fig. 7.41:** Dense echoes in the uterus from calcifications resulting from fibroids.

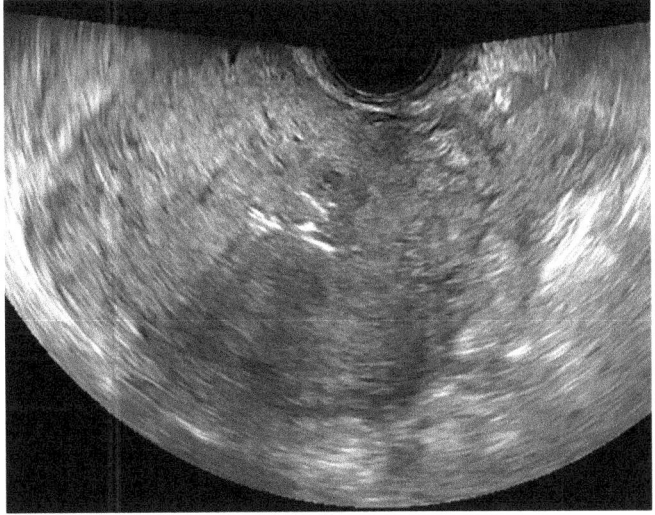

**Fig. 7.42:** Calcific foci seen in the anterior subendometrial area.

The ultrasound findings are:
- Multiple bright spots
- Blood flow pooling
- Probe tenderness
- Evaluate again after antibiotics and anti-inflammatory drugs
- Fluid in endometrial cavity
- Fluid in pouch of Douglas.

## Endometrium

### Endometritis (Fig. 7.43)

- Inflammation of endometrium.
- Seen in patient who had undergone D&C, have/had intrauterine device (IUD), postpartum, and in patient of PID.
- Mycobacterium tuberculosis is also a common cause of chronic endometrial infection.

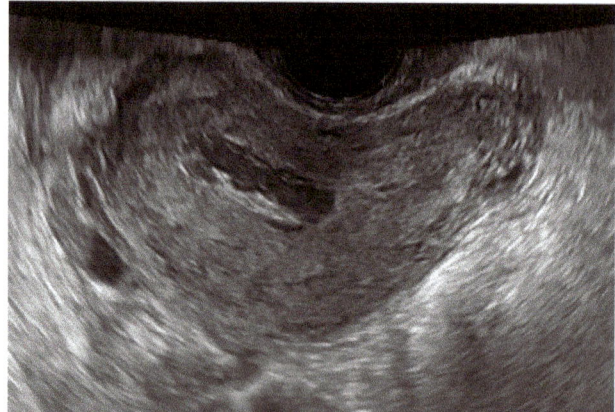

**Fig. 7.43:** Echogenic irregular endometrium because of endometritis.

USG features:
- Increased echogenicity, thickness, vascularity of endometrium and inner myometrium.
- Hyperechoic bridges within the uterine cavity.
- Small amount of fluid in endometrial cavity.
- On CD in acute-stage shows low to moderate RI (RI = 0.50 ± 0.08). In chronic stage shows high resistance flow. In case of irreversible tissue damage shows absence of blood flow.

## Endometrial Hyperplasia (Figs 7.44 to 7.58)

Endometrial thickness >14 mm in perimenopausal.

Endometrial thickness > 4 mm in postmenopausal patient caused by estrogen stimulation.

*USG features:* Thick, inhomogeneous endometrium with small cysts. On CD peripheral blood supply by regular separated vessels is typical shows RI > 0.50. In case of suspicion of malignancy should perform power Doppler and 3 DPD examination to check vascularization which is irregular in case of endometrial carcinoma.

## Endometrial Polyps (Figs 7.59 to 7.65)

Polyps are solitary or multiple, soft, sessile and pedunculated tumors containing hyperplastic endometrium usually asymptomatic. Usually asymptomatic, sometimes present with bleeding, infertility, infection, endometriosis or pain.

USG findings:
- Diffuse or local thickening of endometrium (secretory phase).
- Best visualized during early proliferative phase of menstrual cycle or in secretory phase when surrounded by anechoic fluid (sonohysterography).

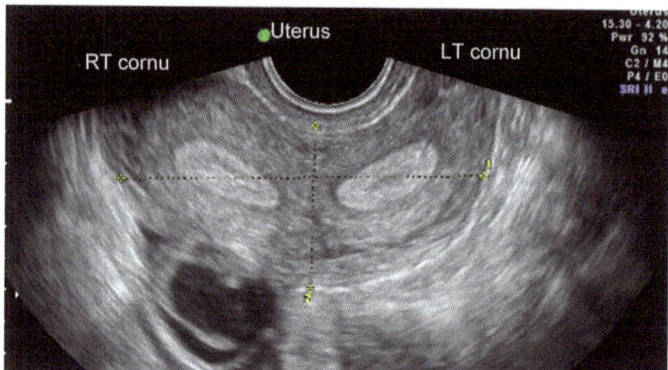

**Fig. 7.44:** Thickened endometrium in septate uterus.

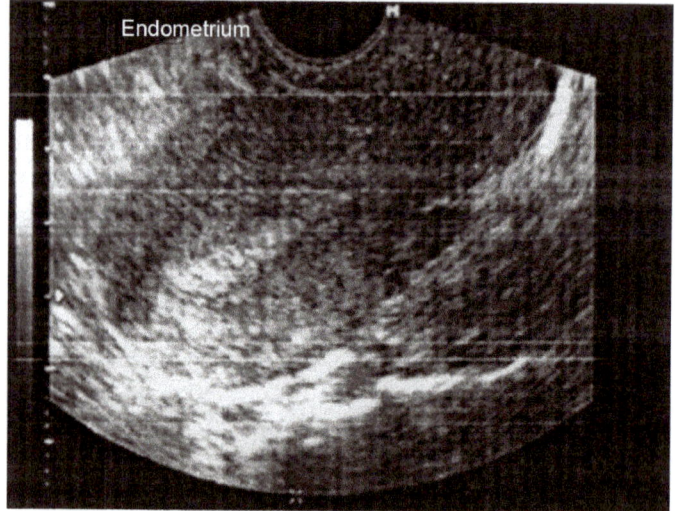

**Fig. 7.45:** Thick endometrium (12–13) seen in a patient bleeding for 12 days.

Uterine Disorders

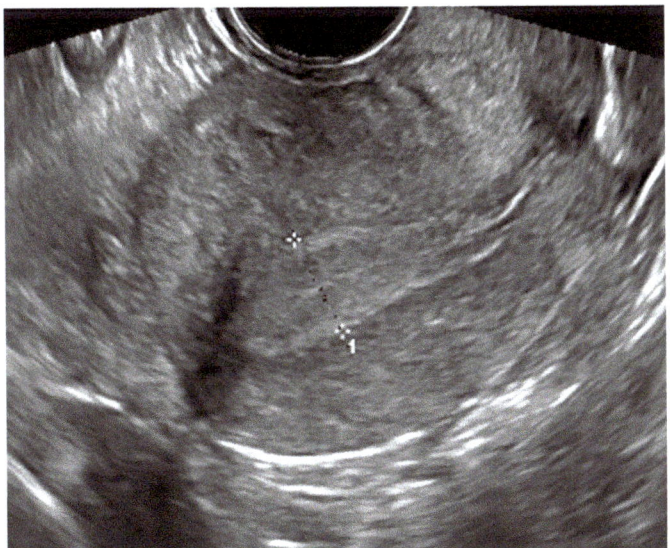

**Fig. 7.46:** Homogeneously thick endometrium (16 mm).

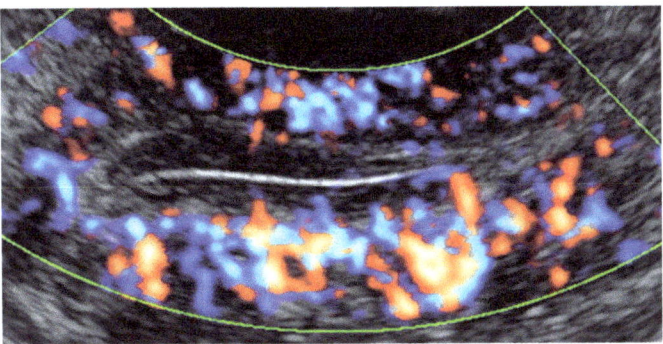

**Fig. 7.47:** Thickened endometrium with moderate endometrial and subendometrial vascularity.

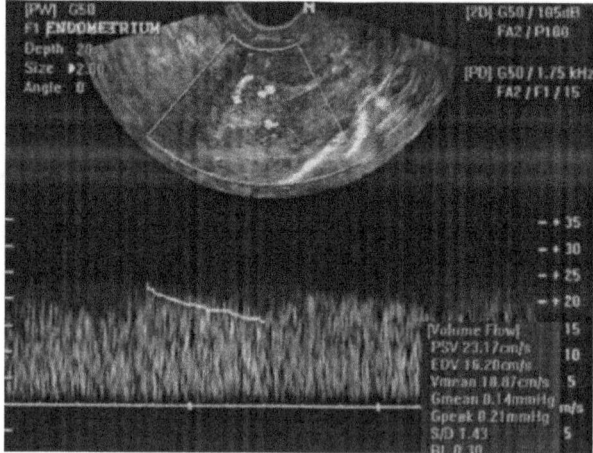

**Fig. 7.48:** Flow velocity waveform shows a low impedance flow with a RI of 0.39.

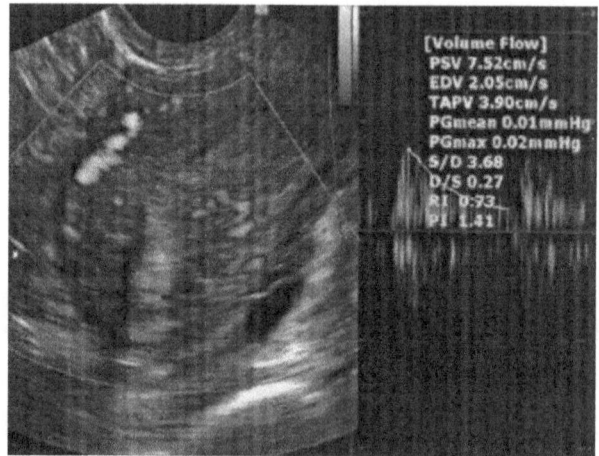

**Fig. 7.49:** Thick endometrium showing a high impedance flow with a RI of 0.73.

Uterine Disorders

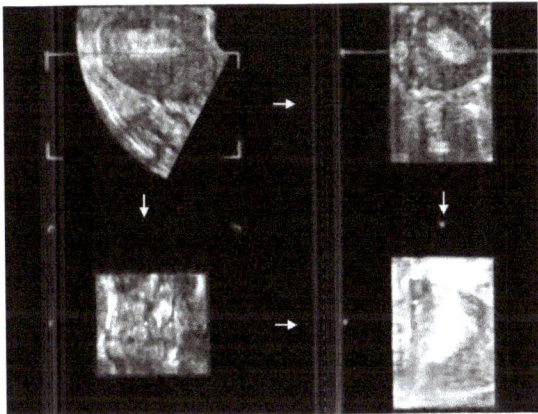

**Fig. 7.50:** The same as seen on 3D reconstruction.

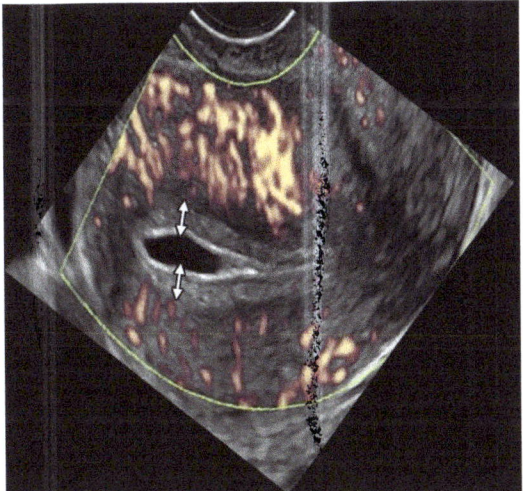

**Fig. 7.51:** Thick endometrium with fluid collection. Exclude the collection from the measurement.

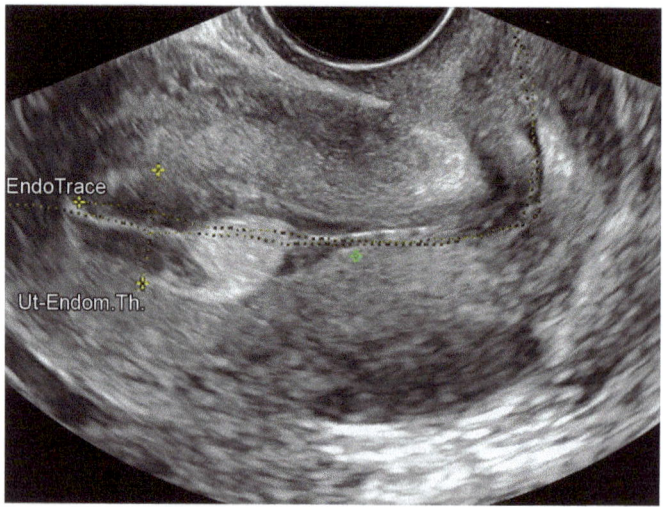

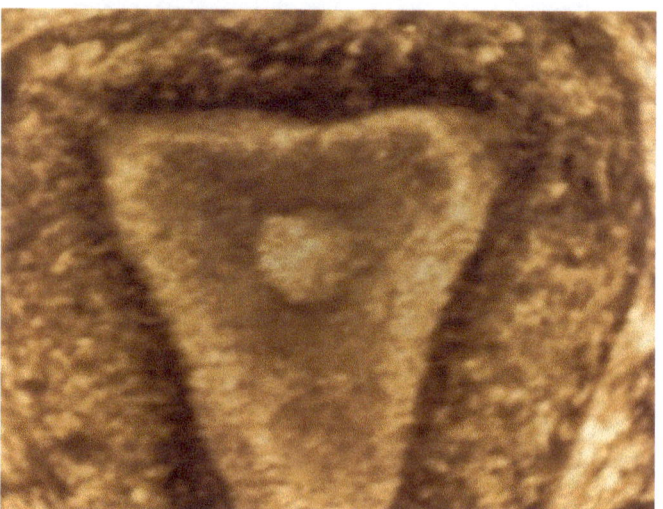

**Fig. 7.52:** Thick endometrium with a mass in the uterine cavity.

Uterine Disorders

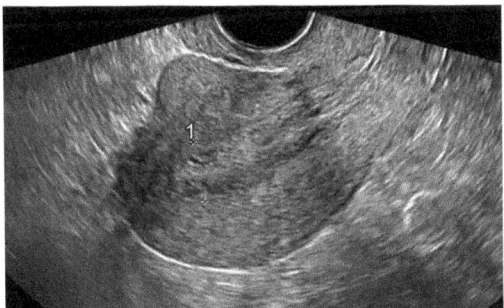

**Fig. 7.53:** Thick endometrium with multiple thin-walled clear cystic spaces.

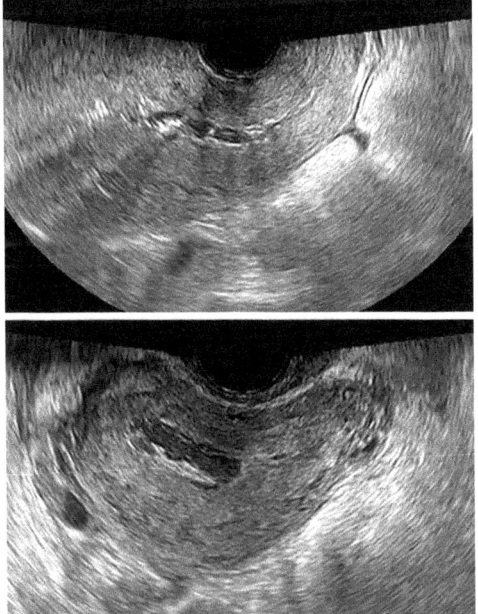

**Fig. 7.54:** Irregularly thickened endometrium in a postmenopausal bleeding patient.

## Ultrasound in Gynecology

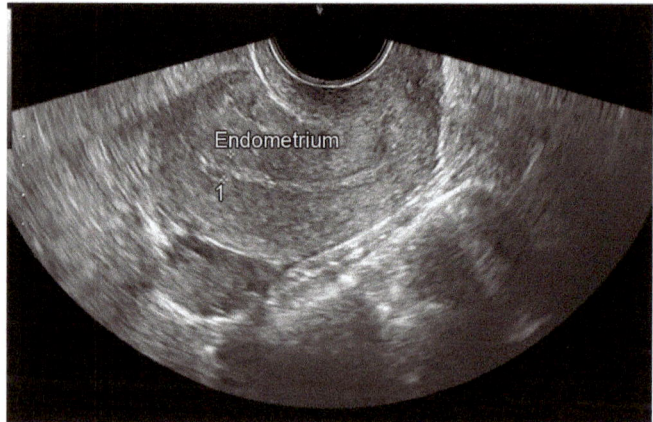

**Fig. 7.55:** Thin endometrium in a postmenopausal patient.

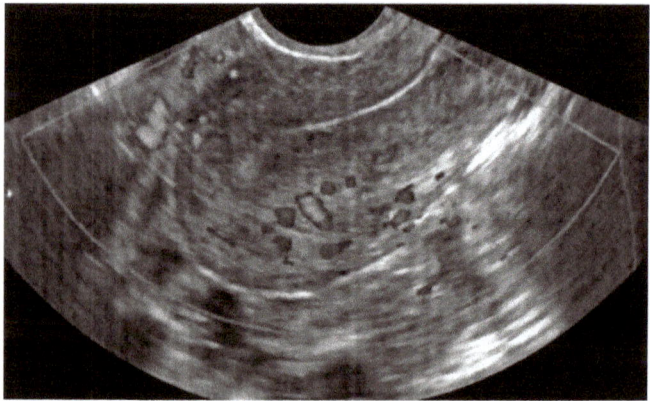

**Fig. 7.56:** The same as seen with color flow mapping.

Uterine Disorders

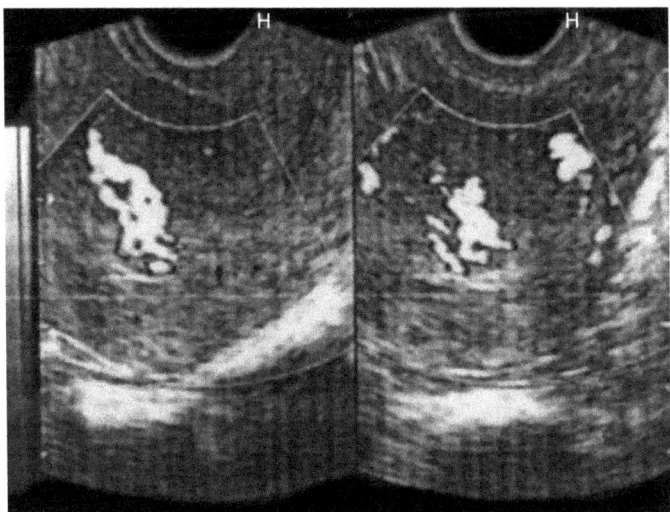

**Fig. 7.57:** Thickened endometrium with moderate subendometrial flow.

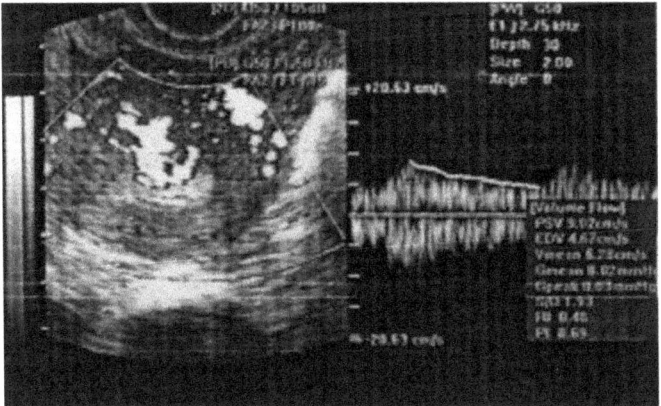

**Fig. 7.58:** On duplex Doppler evaluation the arterial flow velocity waveform shows a low impedance flow.

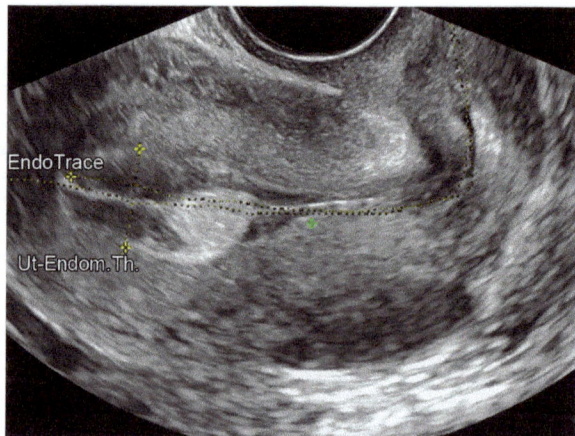

**Fig. 7.59:** Endometrial polyp causing a focal endometrial thickening in a patient of intermenstrual spotting.

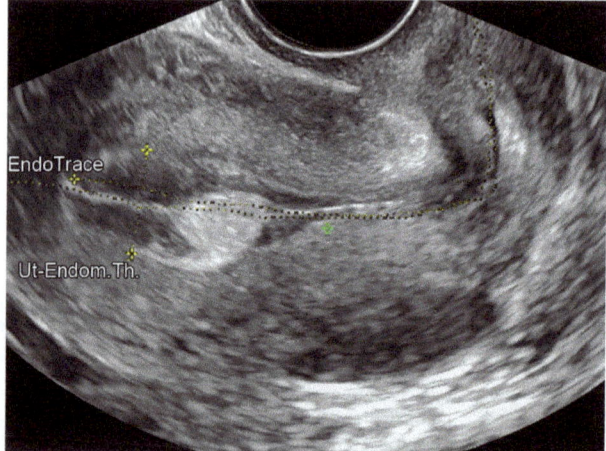

**Fig. 7.60:** Patient of menometrorrhagia with an echogenic endometrial polyp. Note that the interface between the endometrium and the myometrium is preserved.

Uterine Disorders

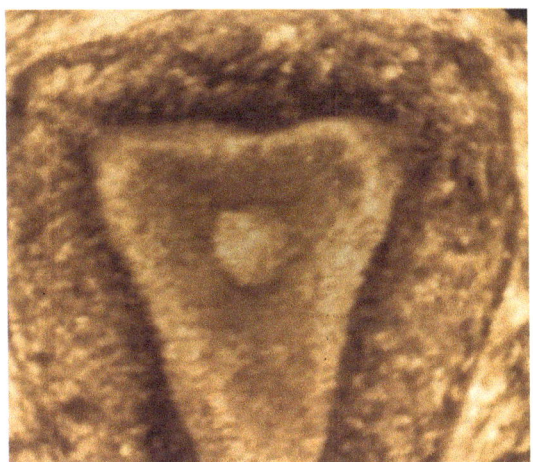

**Fig. 7.61:** Endometrial polyp as seen on 3D.

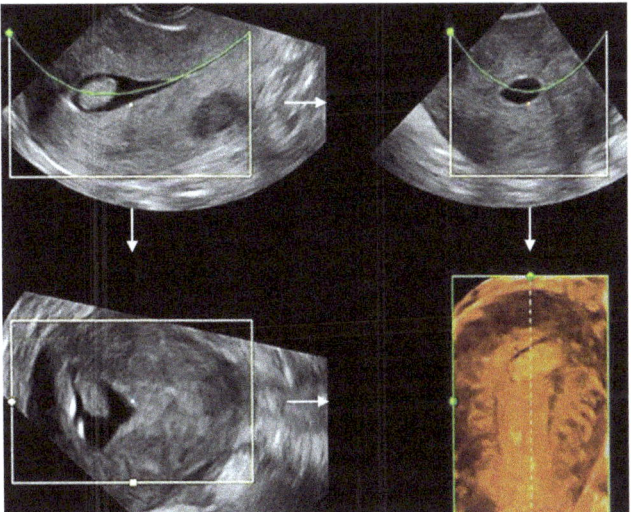

**Fig. 7.62:** Endometrial polyp in posterior wall with fluid collection.

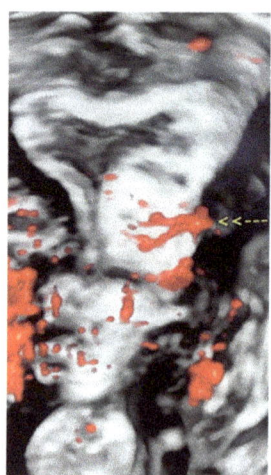

**Fig. 7.63:** The same with color flow mapping.

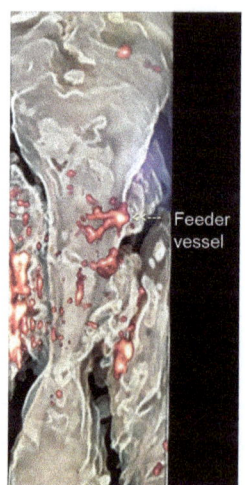

**Fig. 7.64:** Polyp showing pedicle in posterior wall which is vascular.

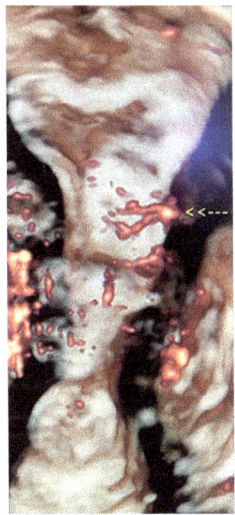

**Fig. 7.65:** Polyp as seen on 3D.

- On CD feeding arteries can be seen, originating from terminal branch of uterine arteries RI 0.45.
- On 3D coronal imaging provides an opportunity to delineate the polyp more accurately because entire endometrial cavity can be seen plane.

### Endometrial Carcinoma (Figs 7.66 to 7.69)

Most common gynecological malignancy and in postmenopausal patients.
*Symptoms*: Postmenopausal bleeding
*Risk factors*: DM, HTN, obesity, plus multiparity, etc.
*USG features*:
- Thickened endometrium >4 mm, inhomogeneous, hyperechoic, with loss of subendometrial halo if there is a myometrial invasion.

- On CD typical sign is neovascularization. Low vascular resistance RI 0.42 ± 0.02.
- On 3D ultrasound endometrium volume >13 mm.
- 3DPD shows randomly dispersed vessels with irregular branching and arborization within the myometrium.

### *Endometrial Fluid*

Fluid within the endometrial cavity is seen in both normal and pathological conditions. In women in the menstrual

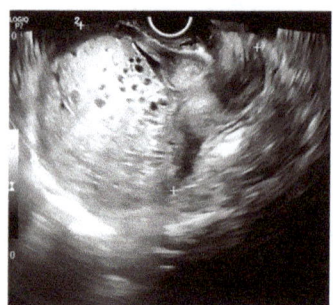

**Fig. 7.66:** Thickened inhomogeneous endometrium with multiple interspersed cystic spaces.

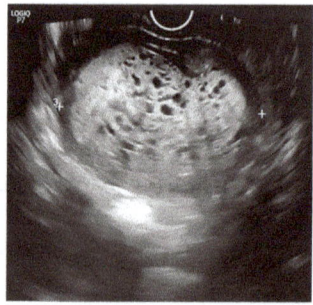

**Fig. 7.67:** Thickened endometrium with multiple cystic spaces.

Uterine Disorders

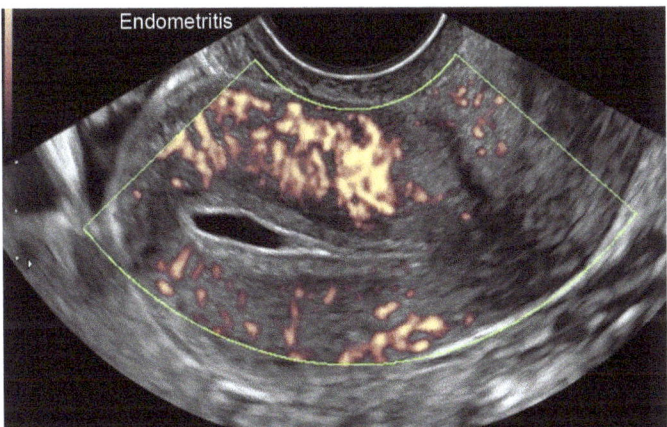

**Fig. 7.68:** Thickened endometrium with a fluid collection and a loss of the endometrial-myometrial interface at the posterior aspect.

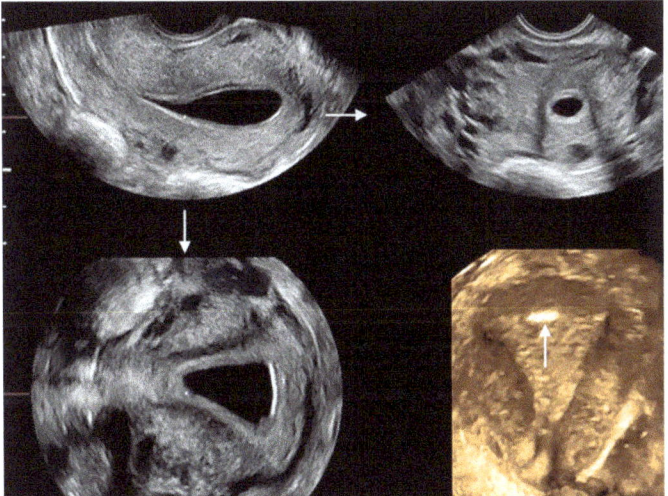

**Fig. 7.69:** Fluid within the cavity with a focal echogenic area.

phase of their cycle, a tiny amount of fluid is a normal finding. Fluid within the endometrium is also seen in normal early pregnancy and abnormal pregnancy (missed abortion, ectopic pregnancy, and molar pregnancy). Other causes of endometrial fluid include infection and obstruction. In older patients, fluid can be secondary to malignancy (uterine, cervical, tubal, or ovarian); however, cervical stenosis of a benign etiology (especially in women who previously had children or instrumentation) is more common. The presence of fever in a woman with a fluid collection suggests pyometra.

### *Intrauterine Contraception Devices (Figs. 7.70 to 7.75)*

Another cause of bright reflectors within the uterus is intrauterine contraceptive devices. Ultrasound is helpful in locating the intrauterine contraceptive device when the string

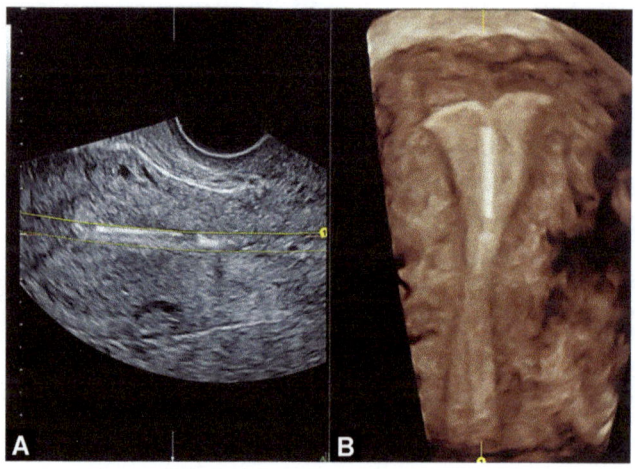

**Figs. 7.70A and B:** IUCD in the uterine corpus.

## Uterine Disorders

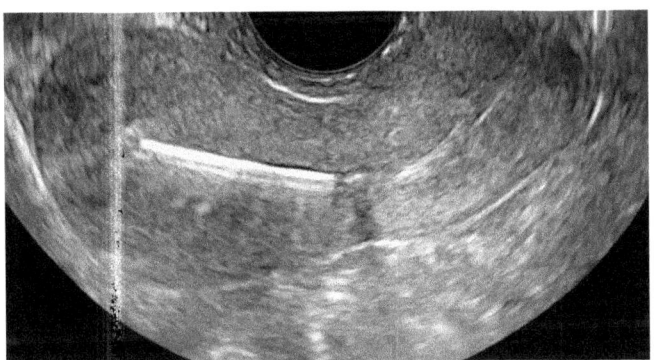

**Fig. 7.71:** Intrauterine contraceptive device seen in the uterine fundus.

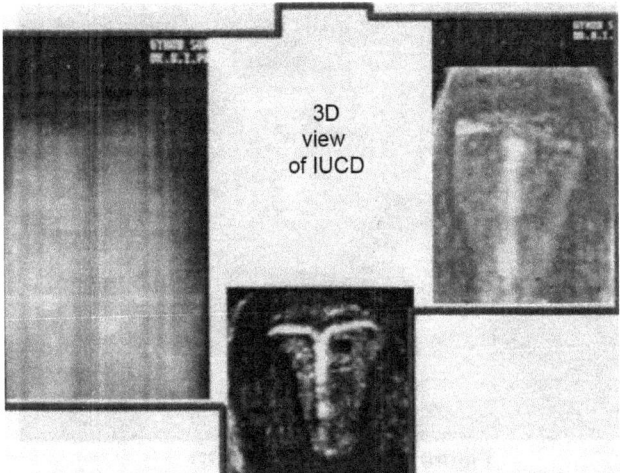

**Fig. 7.72:** 3D for an intrauterine contraceptive device (IUCD) in the cavity.

**138** Ultrasound in Gynecology

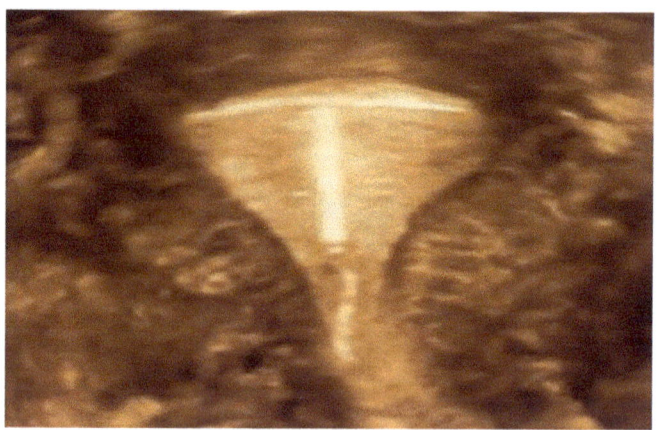

**Fig. 7.73:** Same IUCD as seen on 3D.

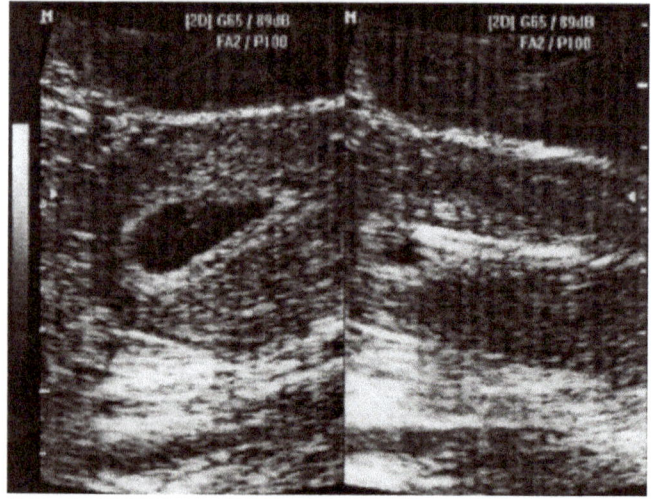

**Fig. 7.74:** IUCD with pregnancy as seen on 2D.

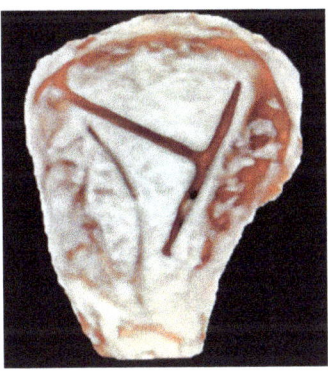

**Fig. 7.75:** With ease on a 3D scan one can see the position of the IUCD and pregnancy.

cannot be felt. Ultrasound is used to precisely locate the position of the intrauterine contraceptive device relative to the endometrial lumen and surrounding myometrium. While 2D user is not able to demonstrate entire IUD, 3D improves detection rate of IUD that have embedded in the myometrium because 3D reconstruct the image in coronal plane, also to visualize complete IUD including shaft and arms.

## Congenital Uterine Anomalies

It results from incomplete fusion of the müllerian ducts in intrauterine life.

According to American Fertility Society classification, their types are divided based on external contour of fundus and the contour of endometrial cavity. Multiplanar imaging and rendered imaging on 3D USG shows both contour and indentation very clearly so 3D USG are best modality to see which is also called virtual hysteroscopy.

# Single Uterine Horn

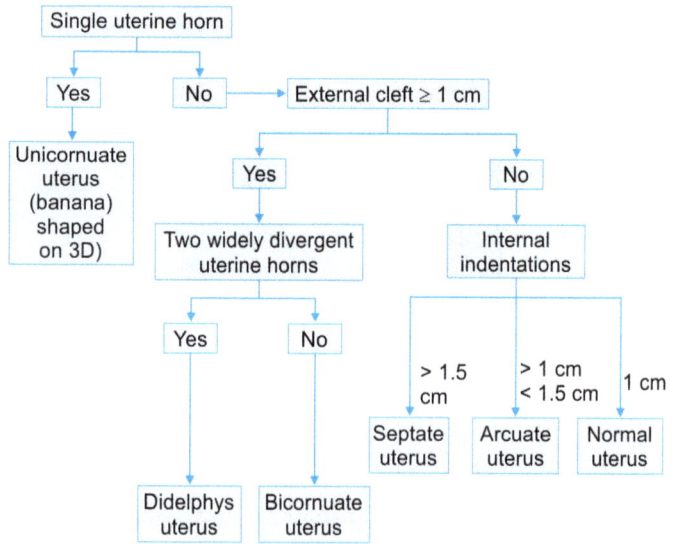

## Uterine Synechiae (Figs. 7.76 and 7.77)

There are fibrotic bands seen across layers of endometrium. They occur due to destruction of basal layer of endometrium due to surgical trauma, e.g. D and C, due to chronic endometritis in PID, and tubercular infection.

On USG:
- Visualized as a hyperechoic bridges, better seen during menstruation.
- Sonohysterography better delineates these adhesions.
- On 3D US shows significant reduction of the endometrial cavity volume.

## Uterine Disorders

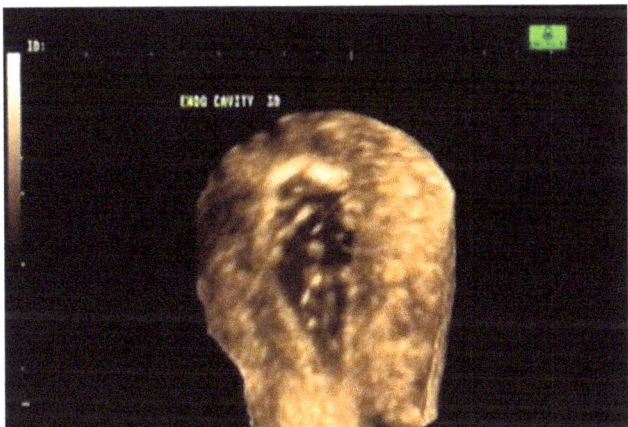

**Fig. 7.76:** Intrauterine adhesions are clearly demarcated after a sonohysterography.

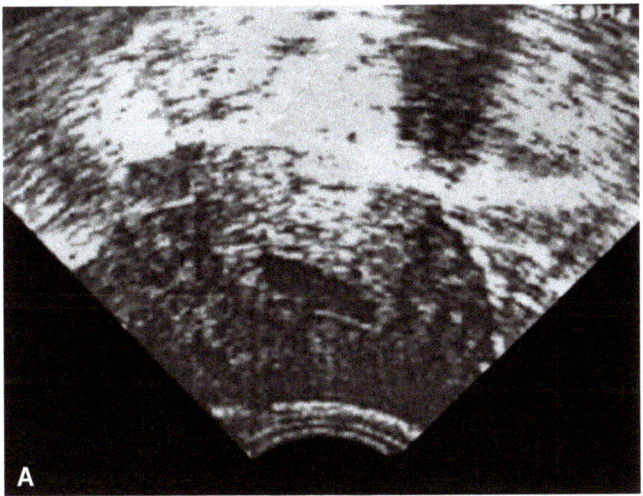

**Fig. 7.77A**

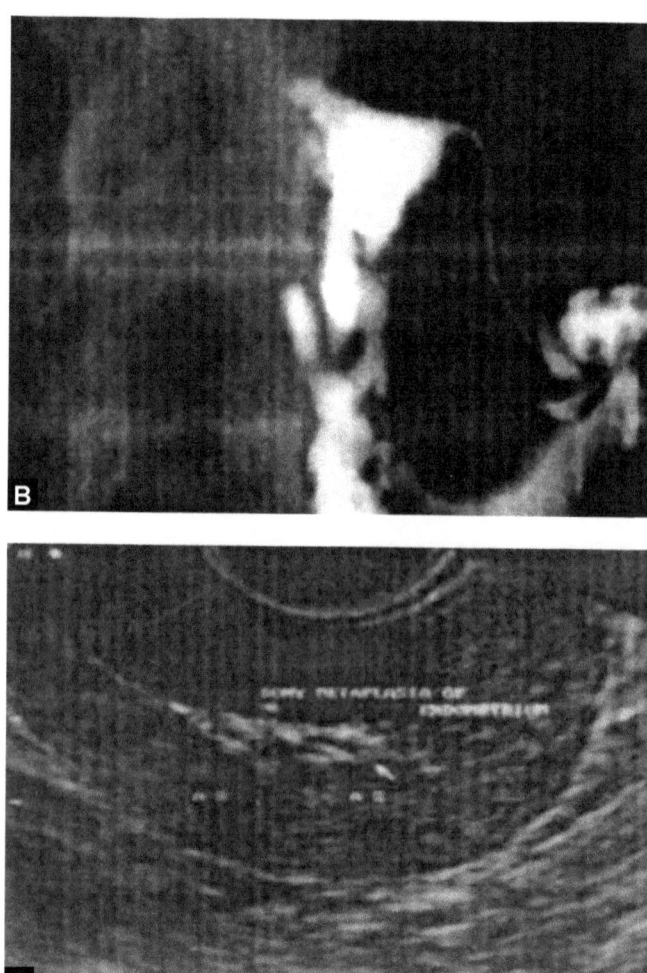

Figs. 7.77B and C

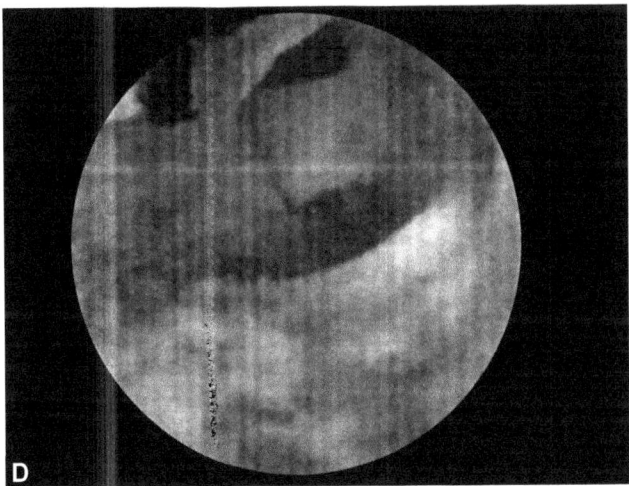

**Figs. 7.77A to D:** Asherman's syndrome as seen on transvaginal scanning, sonohysterography, HSG and hysteroscopy.

## SHAPE AND SIZE (Figs. 7.78 to 7.86)

One can see a small hypoplastic uterus or an uterine anlage in much older females.

## Uterine Cavity Evaluation (Figs. 7.87 to 7.90)

Method which is used for this with an ultrasound called sonohysterography (HyCoSy). It is an USG examination done by using saline contrast media. It is an OPD procedure, less time consuming, cost-effective noninvasive, no anesthesia required, no exposure of radiation, easily reproducible. It can find the cause of underlying problems in case of infertility,

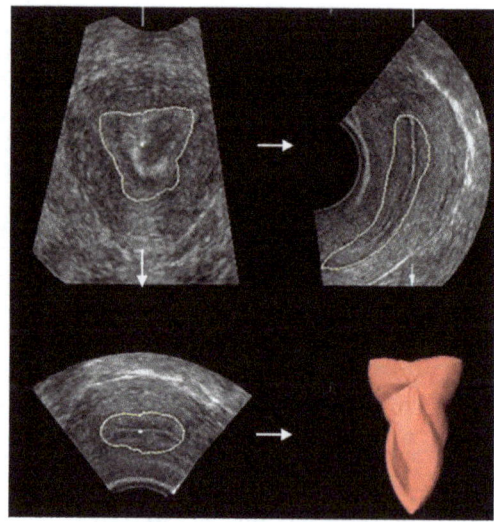

**Fig. 7.78:** A very small uterine anlage in a case of primary amenorrhea.

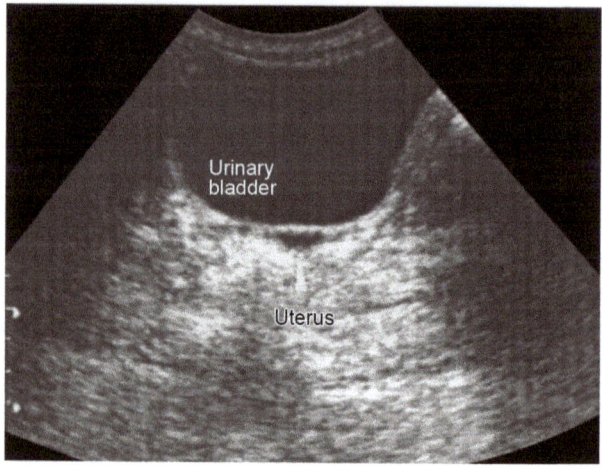

**Fig. 7.79:** Markedly hypoplastic uterus.

Uterine Disorders

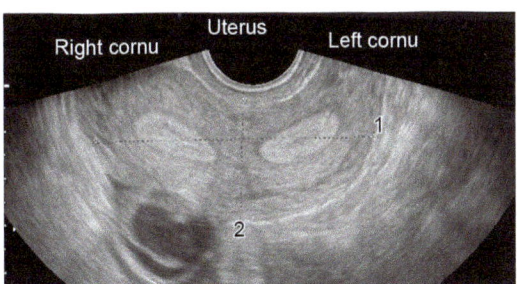

**Fig. 7.80:** Transvaginal scan showing two uteri and a double cervix in the upper portion.

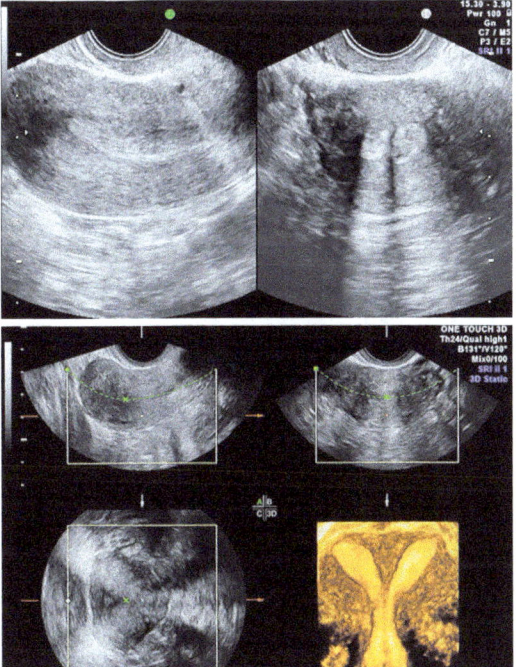

**Fig. 7.81:** Double uterus as seen on 2D.

**146** Ultrasound in Gynecology

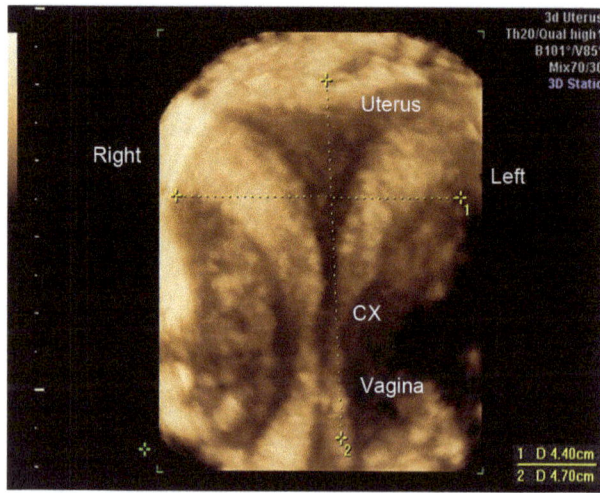

**Fig. 7.82:** Double uterus as seen on 3D.

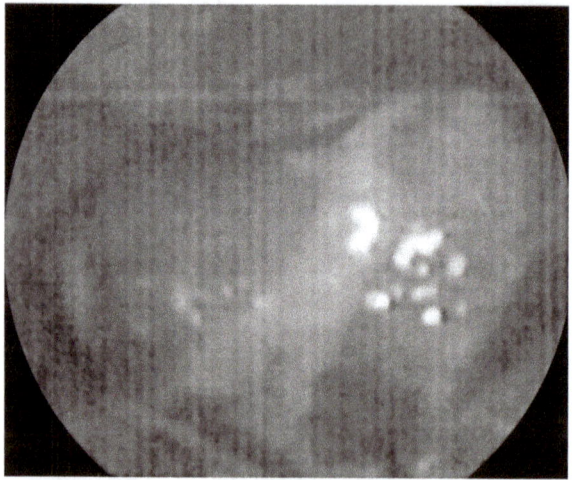

**Fig. 7.83:** Septate uterus as seen on transabdominal and transvaginal ultrasound and confirmed on hysteroscopy.

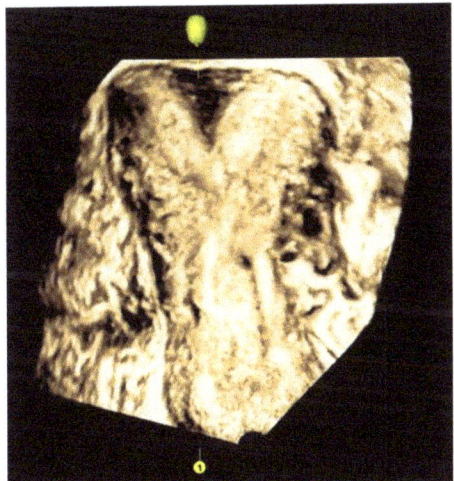

**Fig. 7.84:** Subseptate uterus as seen on TVS.

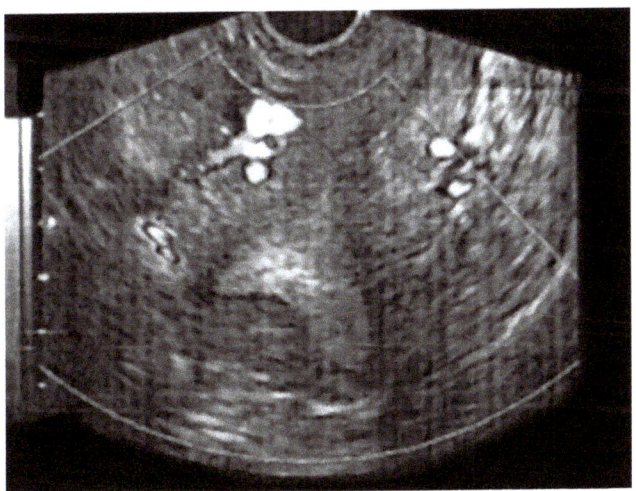

**Fig. 7.85:** Subseptate uterus as seen on TVS and color flow mapping and power angiostudies.

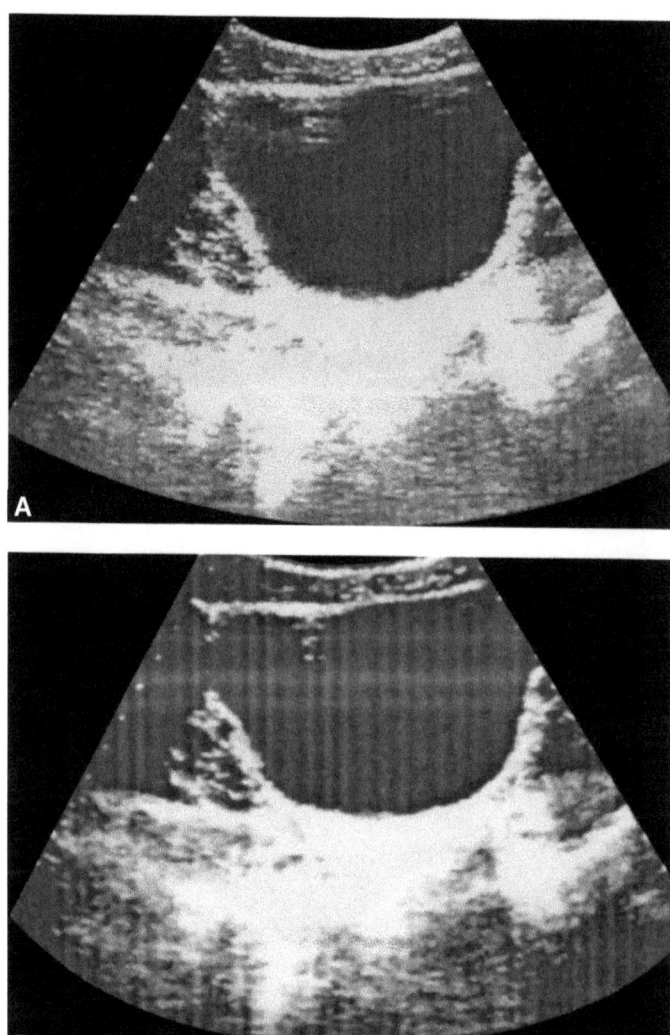

**Figs. 7.86A and B**

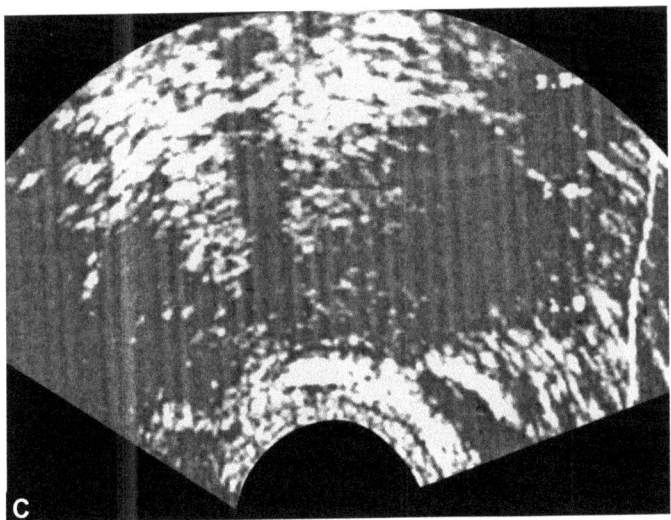
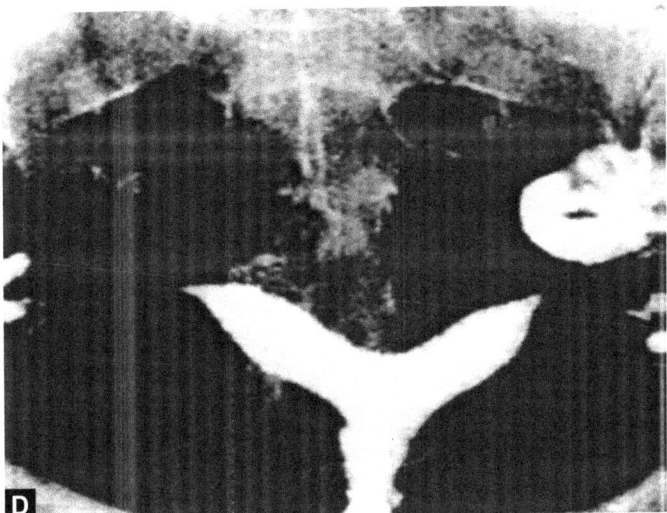

**Figs. 7.86C and D**

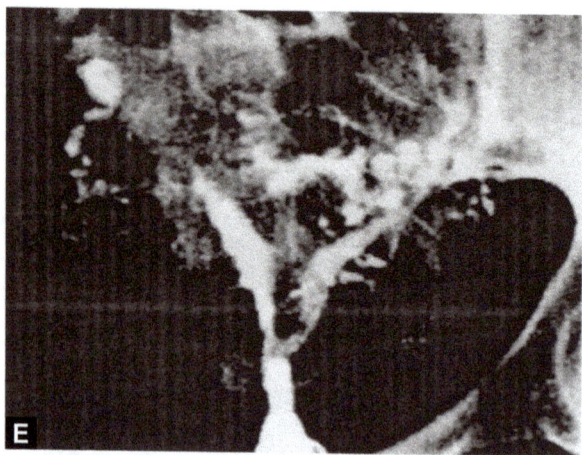

**Figs. 7.86A to E:** Uterine duality as seen on transabdominal and transvaginal ultrasound and confirmed on HSG.

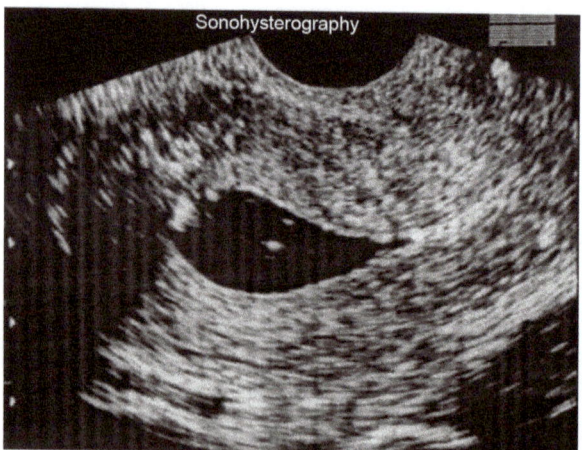

**Fig. 7.87:** Sonohysterography is done by using saline contrast which is pushed through the cervix by a pediatric Foley's or feeding tube under transvaginal scan visualization.

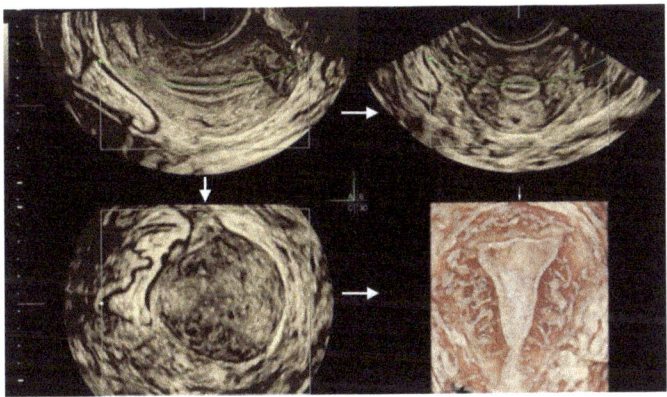

**Fig. 7.88:** This is an excellent, easy, non-invasive, quick and reliable method to evaluate uterine cavity.

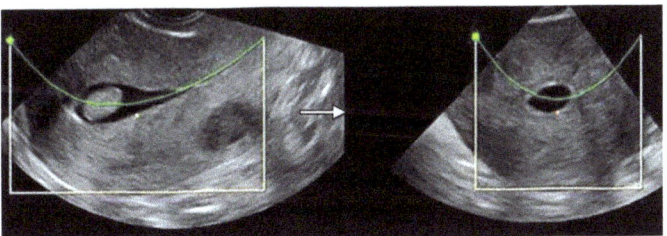

**Fig. 7.89:** Another case of polyp showing so clearly after a sonohysterography.

AUB, pre IVF, malignancy. It is able to detect causes like fibroid, endometrial polyp, Asherman's syndromes, focal lesions, even malignancy. It is done in postmenstrual period.

In this 8F Foley catheter introduced into cervix, balloon is inflated with 1.5-2 mL of distilled water then 5-10 mL of normal saline is injected with 20 mL syringe at the time of scan. Prior to this patient is asked to evacuate the

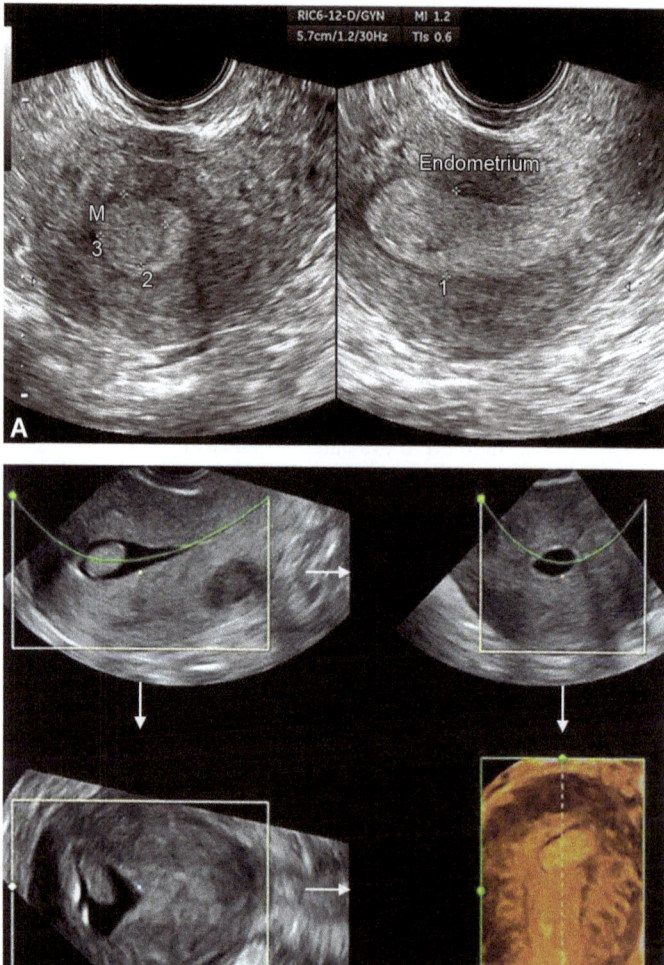

**Figs. 7.90A and B:** Polyp as seen on a transvaginal scan shows up so clearly after a sonohysterography and is excellent to mark the anatomical details.

bladder, baseline scan is done with TVS probe and then after introducing catheter into cavity, again TVS done by using saline as a contrast media.

2D USG shows endometrial pathologies with fluid in situ, we can also take 3D sweep of uterus and can reconstruct in coronal view.

Normal saline gives negative contrast media for intracavitary lesions. We can use positive contrast media, e.g. echovist for this procedure and is called HyCoSy.

# CHAPTER 8

# Ovarian Disorders

The differential diagnosis of an ovarian disorder largely depends on factors such as patient's age, time since last menstrual period, symptoms, pregnancy test result, any prior surgery, and findings on examination. Ovary is the most frequently scanned organ **(Figs. 8.1 to 8.5)** in the female pelvis especially in infertility.

Adnexal masses on ultrasound are labeled as completely cystic, complex (mixed cystic and solid), or solid.

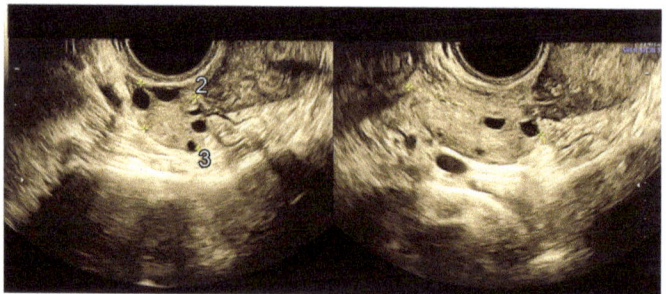

**Fig. 8.1:** Ovary seen in the ovarian fossa the landmarks of which are laterally by internal iliac vessels, medially by uterus and the floor is formed by the obturator internus muscle.

# Ovarian Disorders

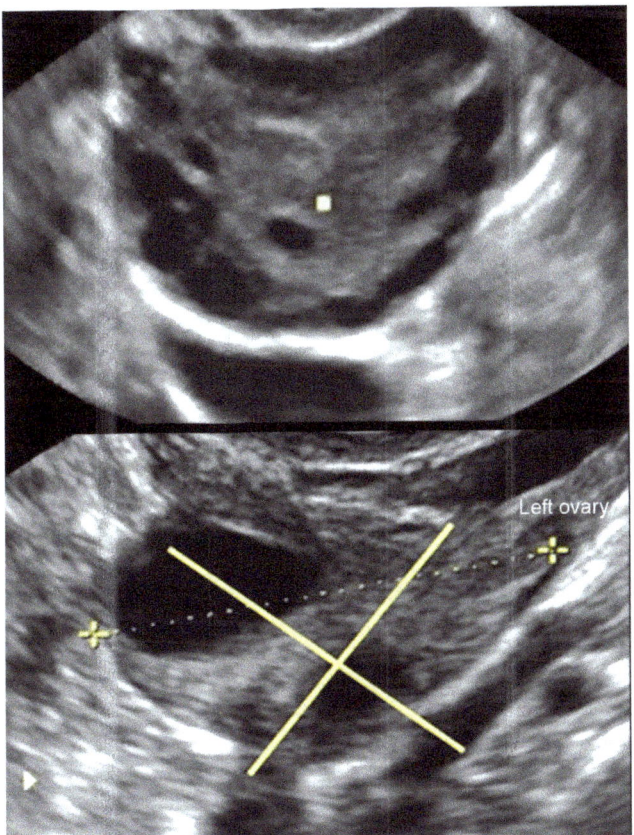

**Fig. 8.2:** Normal ovary as seen on a ultrasound.

## ANECHOIC CYSTS/CYSTIC LESIONS (FIGS 8.6 TO 8.13)

Anechoic cysts are simple cysts, thin-walled, clear fluid filled show distal acoustic enhancement.

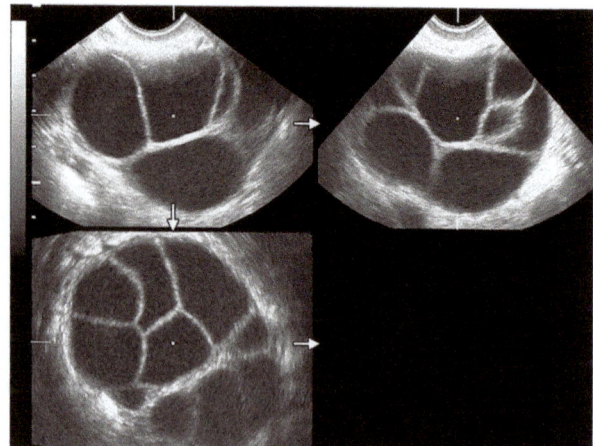

**Fig. 8.3:** Normal ovary as seen on a transvaginal scan showing multiple mature follicles.

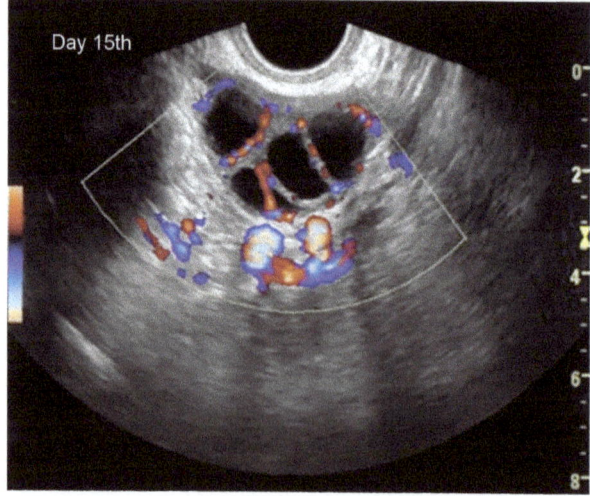

**Fig. 8.4:** Normal ovary with vascular landmark as seen on Sono CT.

# Ovarian Disorders

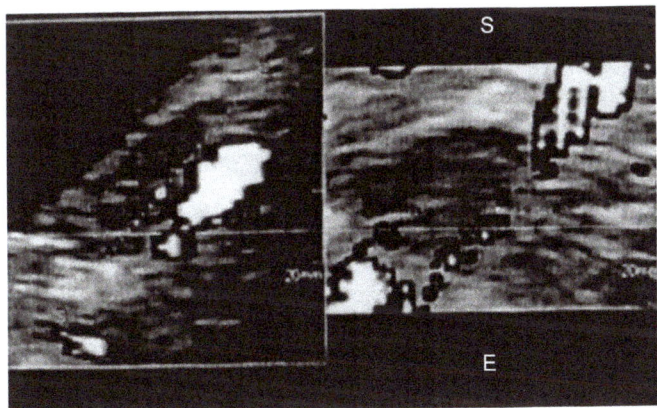

**Fig. 8.5:** Normal ovary with vascular landmark as seen on Sono MR.

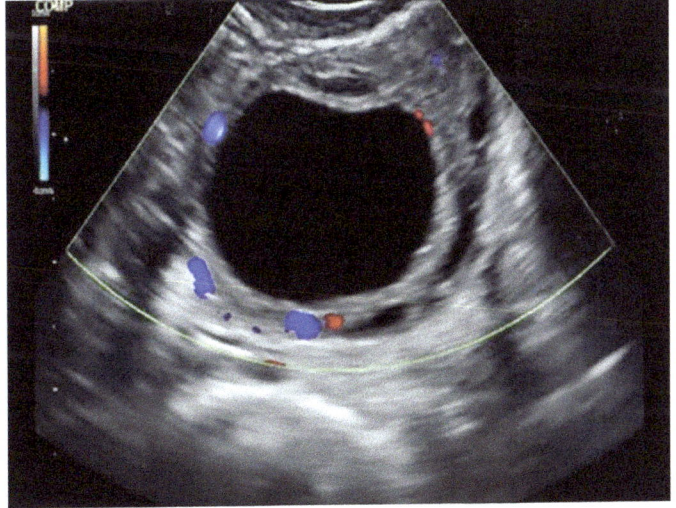

**Fig. 8.6:** Simple anechoic functional cyst.

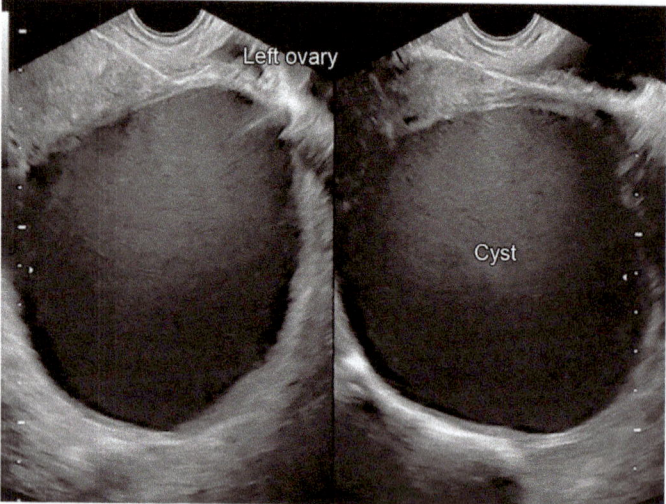

**Fig. 8.7:** Thin-walled cystic area with occasional internal echoes.

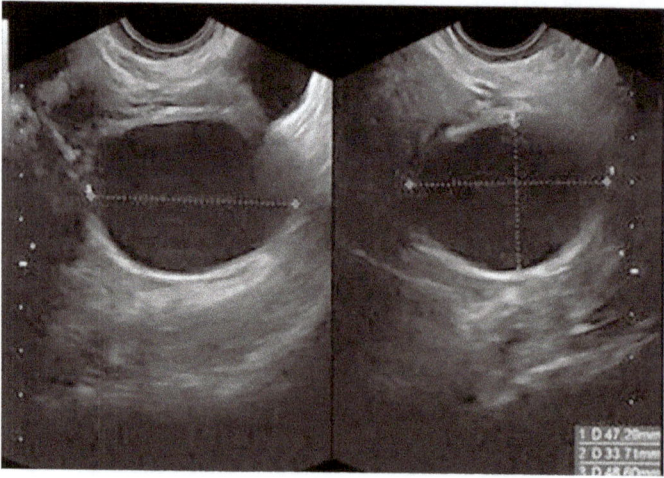

**Fig. 8.8:** Thin-walled clear cystic area in the ovary.

Ovarian Disorders

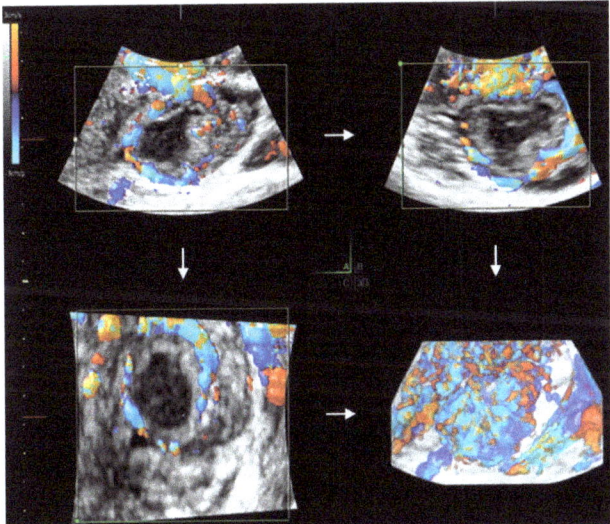

**Fig. 8.9:** Corpus luteum cyst on color flow mapping.

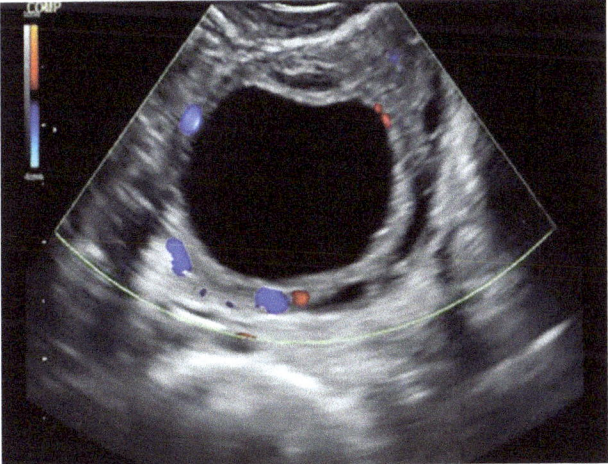

**Fig. 8.10:** Thin-walled clear cystic area.

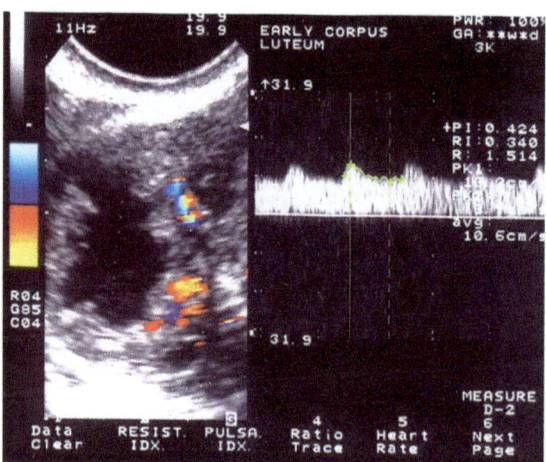

**Fig. 8.11:** Cystic area showing low impedance flow with a RI of 0.47.

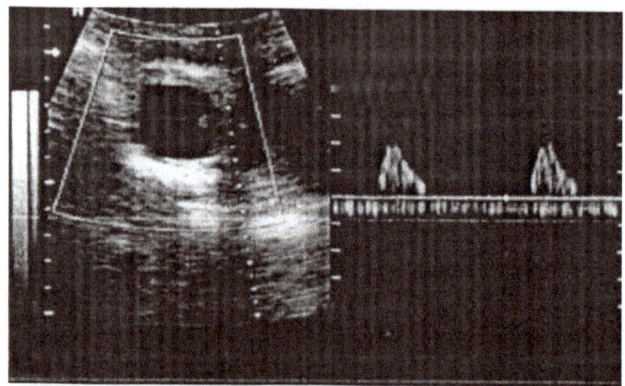

**Fig. 8.12:** Cystic area showing very high impedance flow in ovarian artery.

- *Follicular cyst*: Forms due to failure of mature follicle to rupture at time of ovulation, spontaneously regress,

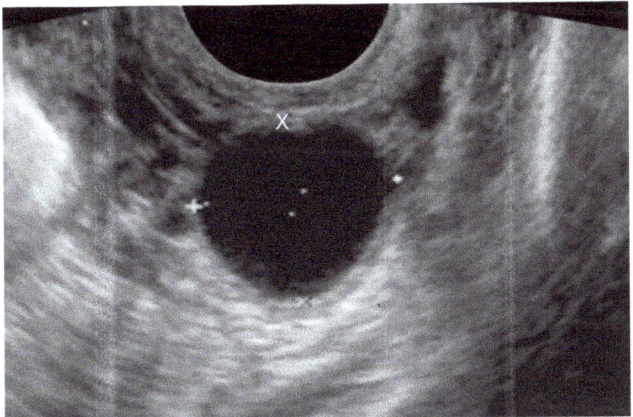

**Fig. 8.13:** Large thin-walled cystic area in the right ovary.

should be followed up, usually small <3 cm but sometimes even up to 10 cm measure.

- *Theca lutein cysts*: Develops due to excessive β-hCG stimulation. Seen in case of ovulation induction and are of GnRH analogs in infertility, in clear pregnancy and multiple pregnancy. Usually bilaterally, spontaneous regress. On USG seen as multicystic thin wall anechoic cyst.
- *Paraovarian cyst*: Arise from remnants of Wolffian duct in *mesovarium, 3–5 cm in diameter* **(Fig. 8.14)**.
- *Hydatid cyst of Morgagni: Arise from fimbriated end of fallopian tube.*

# COMPLEX CYSTS

They contain both fluid and solid areas, can be predominantly solid or cystic.

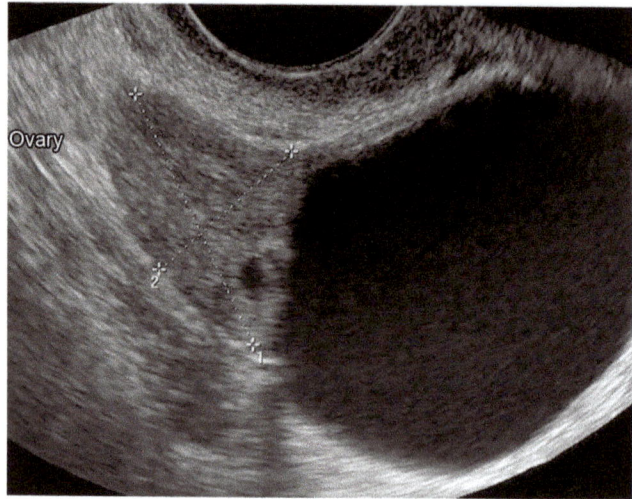

**Fig. 8.14:** Left paraovarian cyst with the left ovary seen separately and the extraovarian cyst which is thin-walled seen separately.

1. *Ovarian endometrioma (chocolate cyst of ovary)* **(Figs 8.15 to 8.17):** On ultrasonography (USG) seen as a single or multicystic ovarian along with low level echoes due to hemorrhage (ground glass appearance) or without solid components. Presence of fluid level or linear bright echogenic foci in wall of cyst favour diagnosis of endometrial cyst.

    On color Doppler (CD) pericystic vascularization at the level of ovarian hilus is typical of endometrioma. It shows no internal vascularity.

2. *Corpus luteum cyst* **(Figs 8.18 to 8.20):** Formed due to continued hemorrhage and collection of blood within corpus luteum, regress within a few weeks.

    On USG complex mass with internal echoes but with enhanced transmission on USG.

## Ovarian Disorders

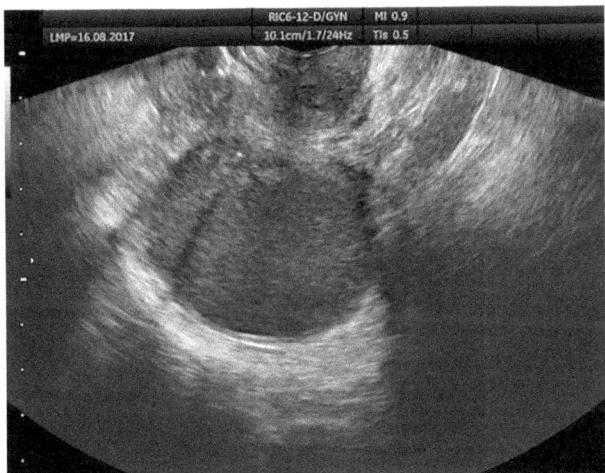

**Fig. 8.15:** Multiple diffuse fine echoes seen in this endometrioma (Ground glass appearance).

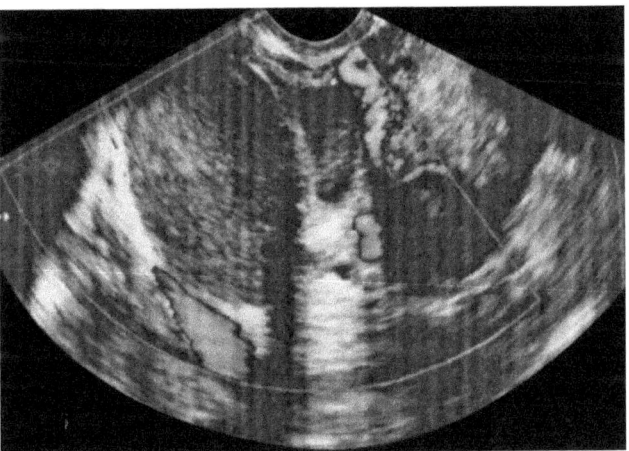

**Fig. 8.16:** Thick-walled endometrioma which is minimally vascular on color flow imaging and power angio studies.

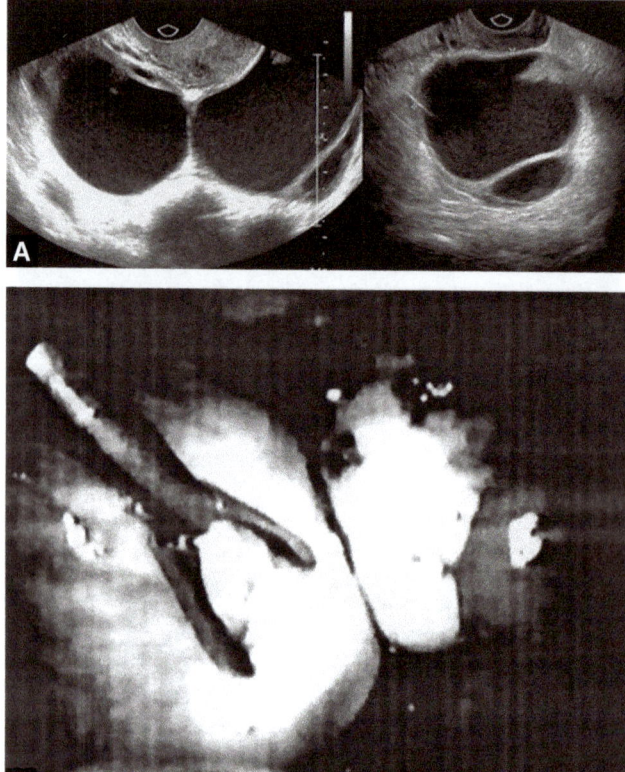

**Figs. 8.17A and B:** Bilateral endometriomas as seen on ultrasound and at laparoscopy.

On CD shows peripheral vascularization (Ring of fire pattern).
3. *Polycystic ovaries* **(Figs. 8.21 and 8.22):** Polycystic ovaries (PCOs) is considered when at least two of following are present (Rotterdam criteria):

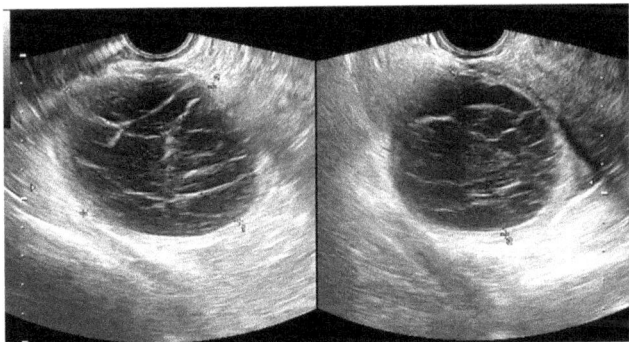

**Fig. 8.18:** Hemorrhagic cyst with dense coarse internal echoes.

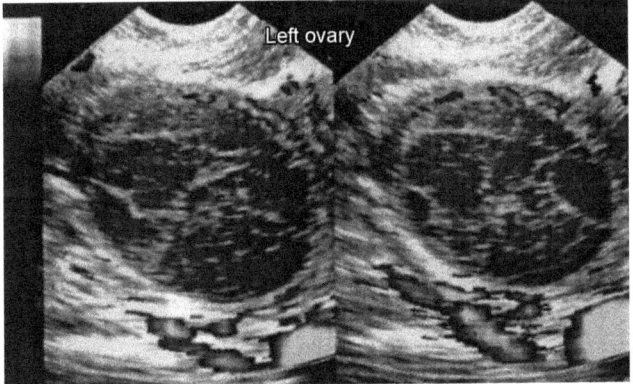

**Fig. 8.19:** The same cystic area as in Figure 8.13 showing a mild rim vascularity.

- Oligoovulation/anovulation
- Hyperandrogenism
- Polycystic ovaries on USG
  ⇒ On USG findings of PCO:
  ⇒ Ovaries length >3.5 mm
  ⇒ Ovarian volume >6.5 cc

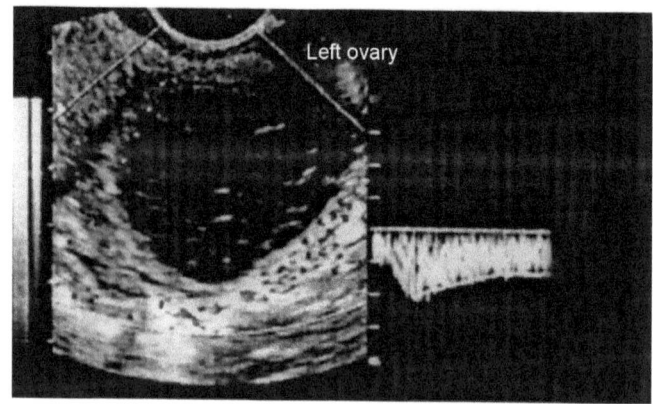

**Fig. 8.20:** On duplex Doppler evaluation the arterial flow velocity waveform shows a mildly impedance flow with a resistive index (RI) of 0.56.

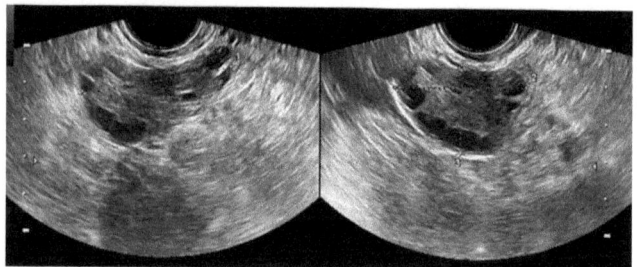

**Fig. 8.21:** Polycystic like ovaries with a dense stroma and multiple thin-walled clear cysts along the periphery.

Multiple follicles (>12 in No) (2-9 mm in diameter) peripherally arranged seen within the cortex (Necklace sign). There is also increased stromal density.

*On CD:* PCO shows stromal flow on baseline scan.

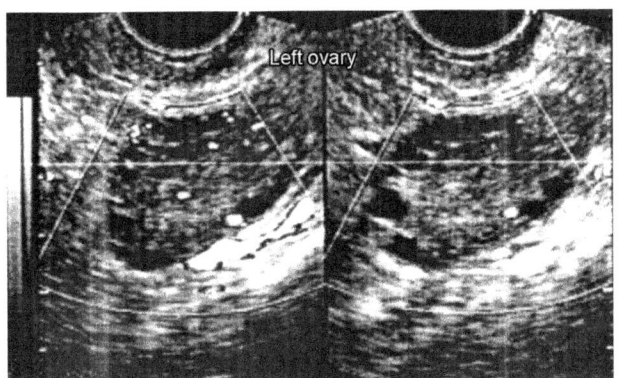

**Fig. 8.22:** Polycystic ovaries with intraovarian blood flow.

On PD all stromal vessels show RI 0.50–0.50. suggestive of high LH level reflections. In PCO ovaries uterine artery show high PI because of high androgen levels in these patients.

4. *Tubo-ovarian complex/Abscess* (**Figs. 8.23 and 8.24**): It forms when inflammatory process involve the ovary almost secondary to salpingitis caused by PID of bacterial origin.
   *On USG:* Seen as inhomogeneous mass within the ovary and tube seen engulfed within it.

5. *Dermoid cyst:* Also called mature cystic teratoma of ovary. Most common benign germ cell tumor of ovary. Most commonly seen during reproductive age group.
   *On USG:* Appears as a completely cystic mass, cystic mass with echogenic mural nodule (Rokitansky protuberance), fat fluid level, differ bright echoes with or without posterior acoustic shadow (teeth or bone), hyperechoic lines or dots (due to hair). Sometimes appear as complex mass with within internal septations and bright linear echoes (**Figs. 8.25 to 8.32**).

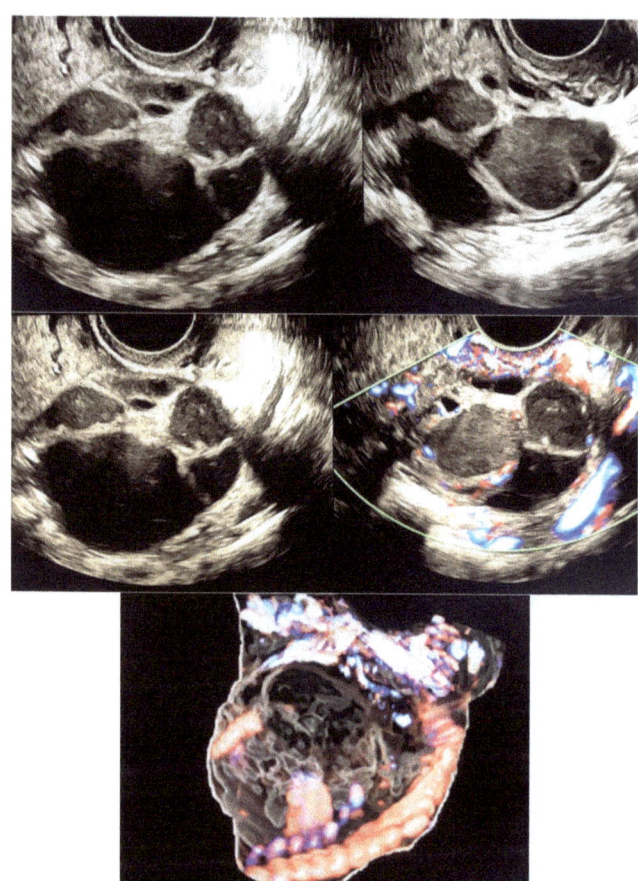

**Fig. 8.23:** Inhomogeneous right adnexal mass.

## OVARIAN NEOPLASM (FIGS 8.33 TO 8.36)

It may be difficult a lot of times to evaluate the cyst contents: fluid, pus, blood or chocolate. Fluid is clear black, blood

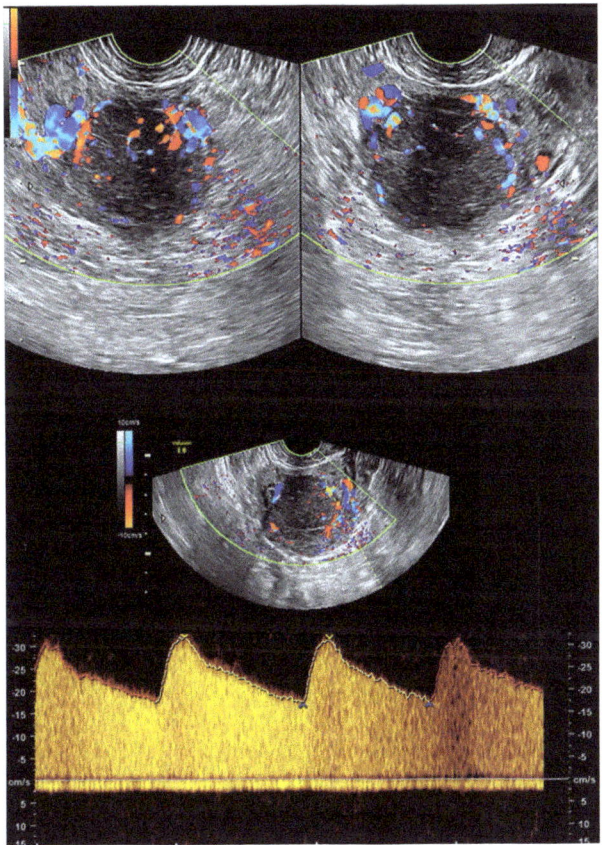

**Fig. 8.24:** Inhomogeneous left adnexal mass with low impedance flow (RI 0.39 suspected malignancy).

shows a reticular pattern which is due to clot formation and retractions, pus usually shows a layering sign and altered blood as in an endometrioma shows classical ground glass appearance with a positive wobble sign.

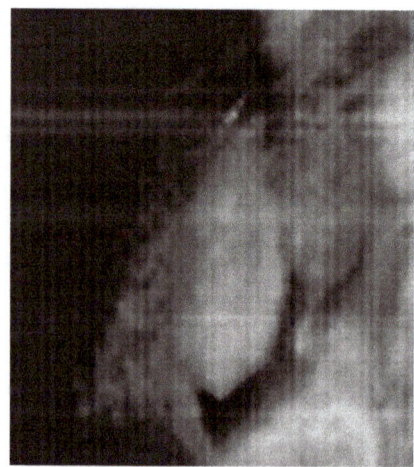

**Fig. 8.25:** Ovarian dermoid as seen on 3D.

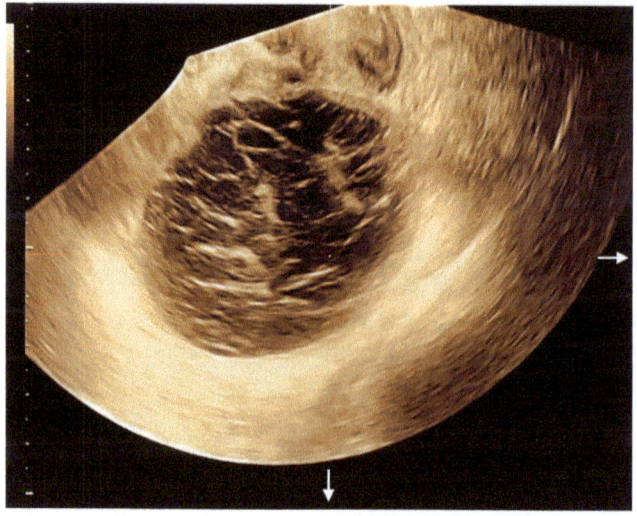

**Fig. 8.26:** Ovarian dermoid may present like this.

Ovarian Disorders

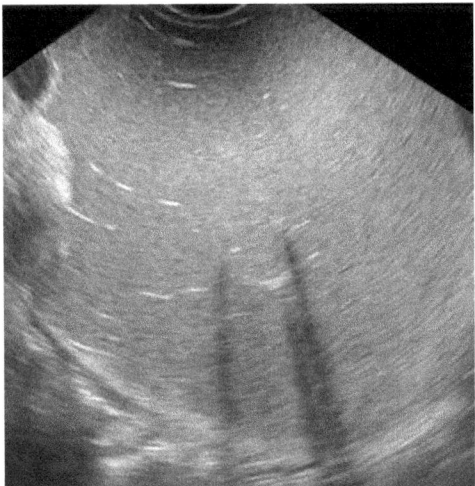

**Fig. 8.27:** Large dermoid with punctate hyperechoic foci.

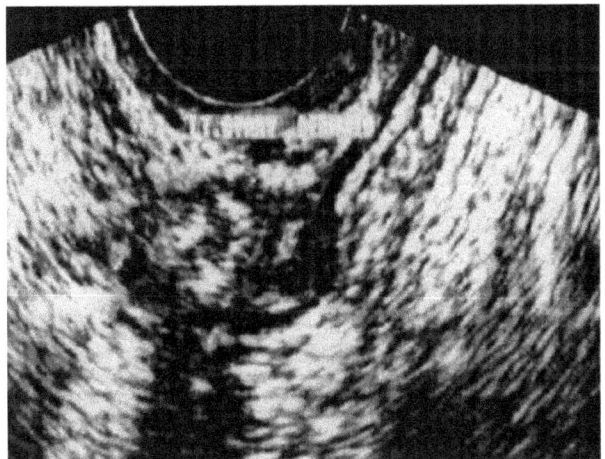

**Fig. 8.28:** Left ovarian dermoid with normal left ovarian tissue seen lateral to it.

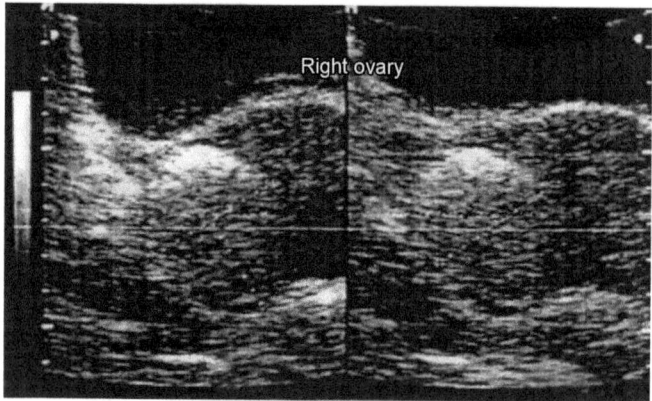

**Fig. 8.29:** Right ovarian dermoid as seen on transabdominal scan.

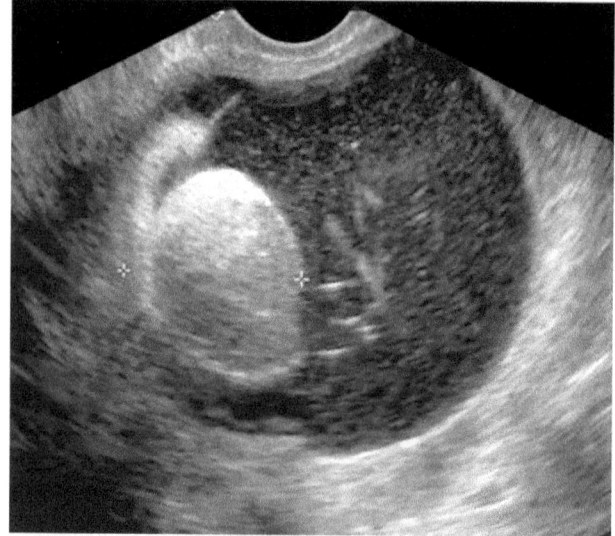

**Fig. 8.30:** Dermoid as seen on transvaginal scan.

Ovarian Disorders

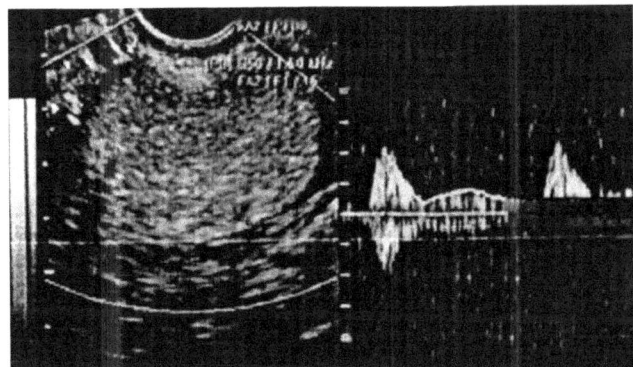

**Fig. 8.31:** Dermoid showing high impedance flow with a RI of 0.88.

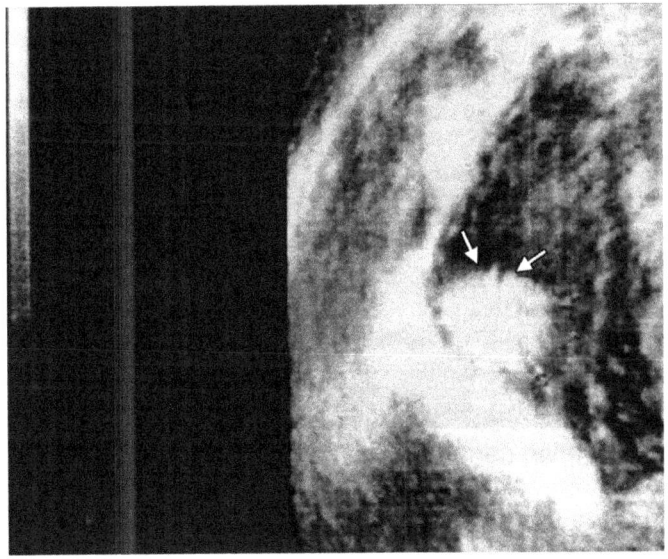

**Fig. 8.32:** Ovarian dermoid as seen on 3D scan.

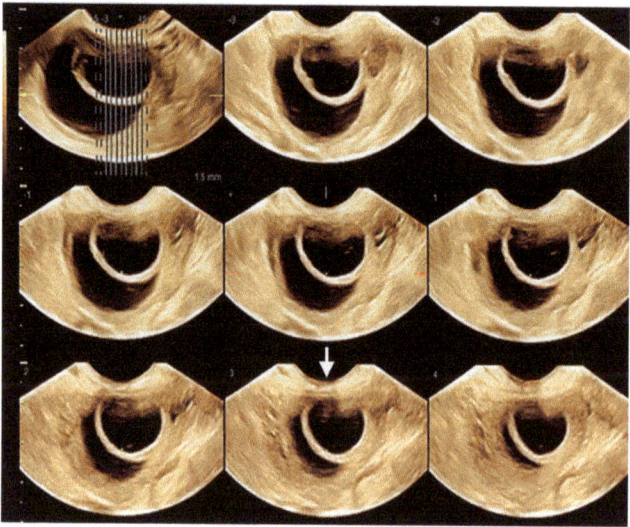

**Fig. 8.33:** Thin-walled clear cystic mass in the left adnexa. Anechoic ovarian mass with multiple thin-septae.

- *Serous cystadenomas*: Most common type of cystic ovarian benign tumor, arises from surface epithelium of ovary most commonly seen in postmenopausal women between 45 and 65 years of age.
  *On USG:* It appears as sharply marginated anechoic mass, usually unilocular, internal thin-walled septations occasionally papillary projection seen, most common in borderline tumor.
  *Serous cystadenocarcinoma:* Usually multilocular contain multiple papillary projections and septations. Echogenic material is occasionally present within loculi.
- *Mucinous cystadenomas:* On USG appear thicker and more numerous septations and contain fine gravity dependent

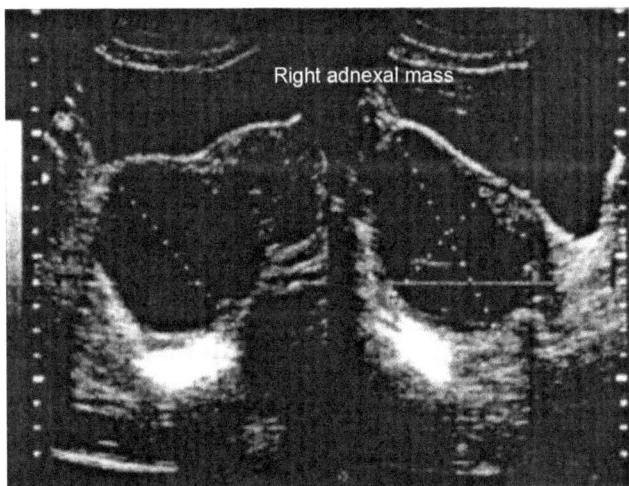

**Fig. 8.34:** Long thin-walled clear cystic masses in the right abdomen.

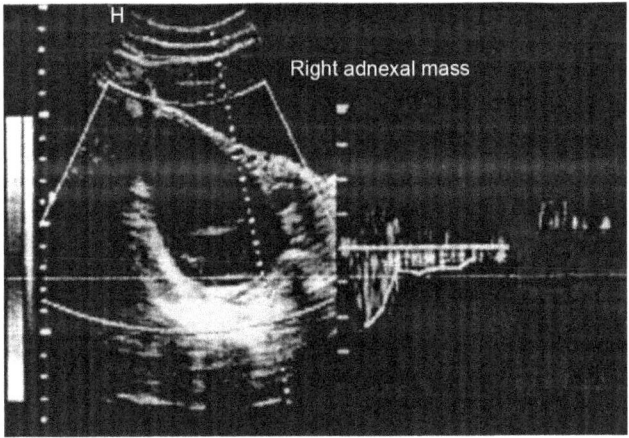

**Fig. 8.35:** Same mass showing high impedance flow with a RI of 0.88.

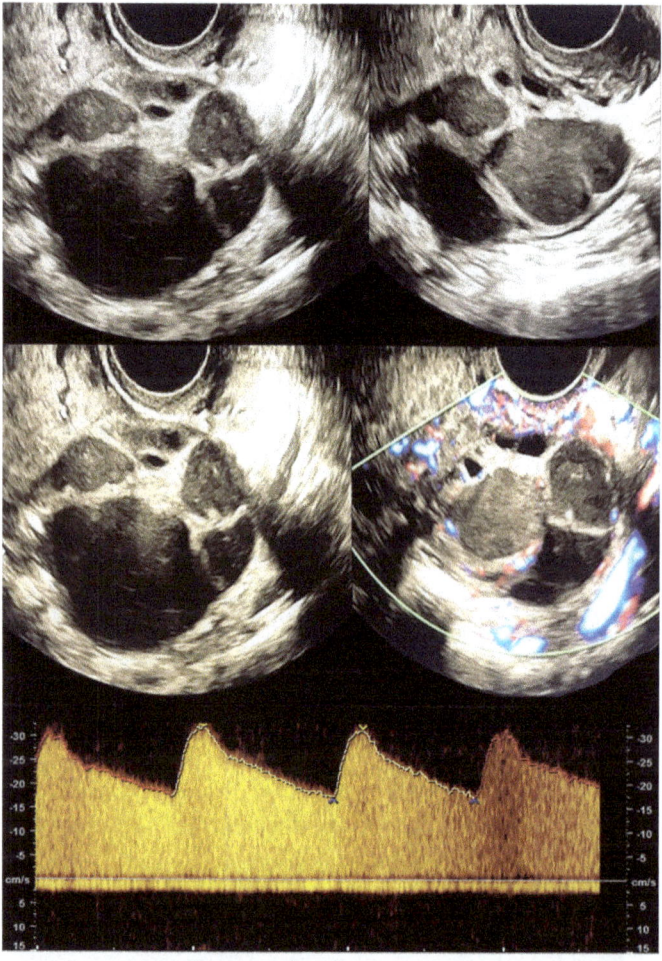

**Fig. 8.36:** Ill-defined mass within the cystic area and coarse internal echoes and large area of solid echoes suspected malignancy.

echoes produced by thick mucinous contrasts. Presence of solid component is seen due to debris, gentle tap on the cyst wall with probe result in movement of debris confirm the diagnoses of pseudomass.

*Mucinous cystadenocarcinomas* appear as large multi-loculated cystic lesions contain echogenic material and papillary excrescences. They have papillary projections less frequently than serous type.

- *Endometrioid tumor*: Second most malignant ovarian epithelial tumor.

  On USG appear as cystic mass containing papillary projection in same case show predominantly solid mass.

## SOLID OVARIAN TUMOR (FIG. 8.37)

Benign solid ovarian tumors are fibroma, thecoma, Brenner tumor.

USG features of fibromas has similar appearance as uterine fibroid with variable attenuation and multiple edge shadows because of chord appearance of tumor.

All malignant arisen neoplasm are solid ovarian mass.

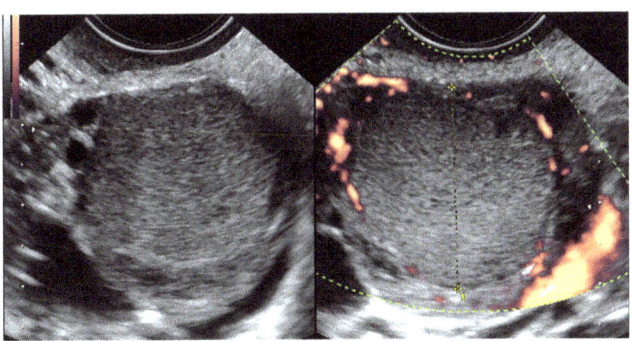

**Fig. 8.37:** Solid right ovarian mass.

## Evaluation of an Ovarian Mass on USG

### Morphologic Parameters

Benign tumor shows unilocular thin smooth wall, clear contents while malignant show thick, irregular walls or septa, multilocular poorly defined borders, usual nodular, solid and echogenic components.

*On color flow mapping:* Benign show peripheral vascularization while malignant show central vascularization.

*On CD:* Malignant tumor b/c of feature of neo vascularization show high velocity, low resistance flow RI < 0.4 and PI 1.

*Arrangement of vessels:* Benign have regularly spread vessels while malignant show randomly dispersed vessels.

*Role of 3D:* It helps in identifying extend of capsular infiltration of tumors, papillary projections and calculating the volume.

*3 DPD:* Shows typical vascularity within microaneurysm, AV shunts, tunnel lakes, dichotomas branching.

# CHAPTER 9

# Miscellaneous Disorders

## CERVICAL DISORDERS (FIGS. 9.1 TO 9.6)

### Nabothian Cysts

Dilated endocervical glands filled with mucus formed due to blockage of cervical glands mouths, as a result of epidermalization.

*On USG:* Appears as anechoic cyst few mm to 4 cm, seen close to cervical canal.

They are of no significance unless infection is present.

### Cervical Fibroid

Benign trauma of smooth muscle origin. In supravaginal portion usually they are interstitial or subperitoneal. In vaginal portion usually pedunculated rarely visible.

*On USG:* Appears as hypoechoic concentric mass, focal area of increased echogenicity suggestive of calcification in fibroid.

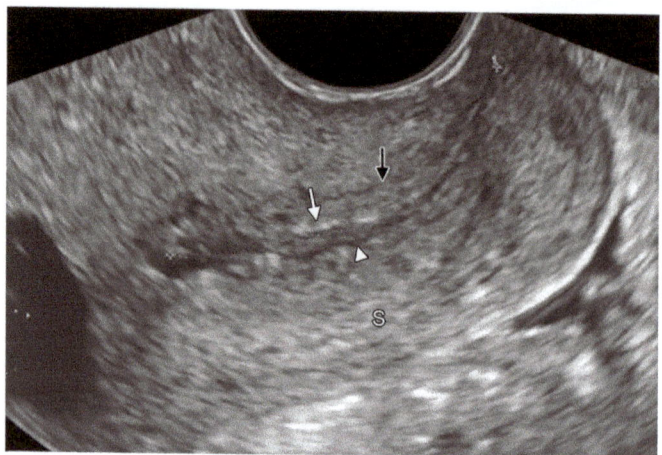

**Fig. 9.1:** Normal cervix seen with the canal and musculature.

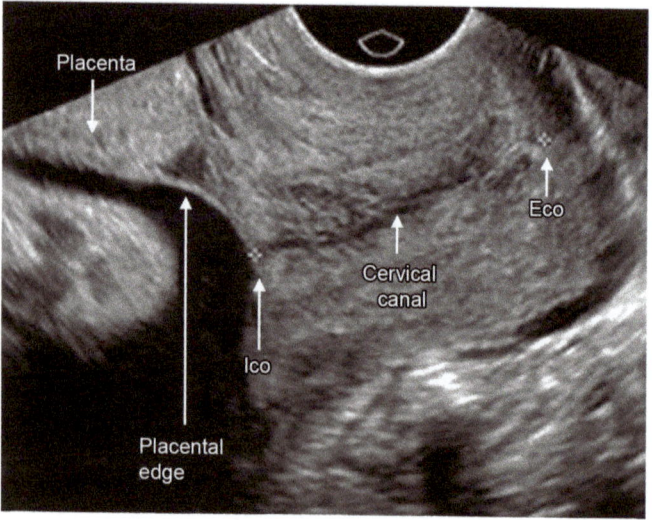

**Fig. 9.2:** Cervical canal with the internal os.

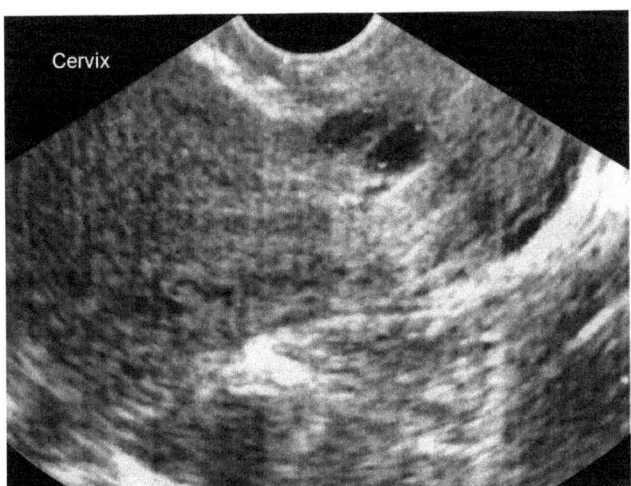

**Fig. 9.3:** Multiple endocervical glands seen in the cervix.

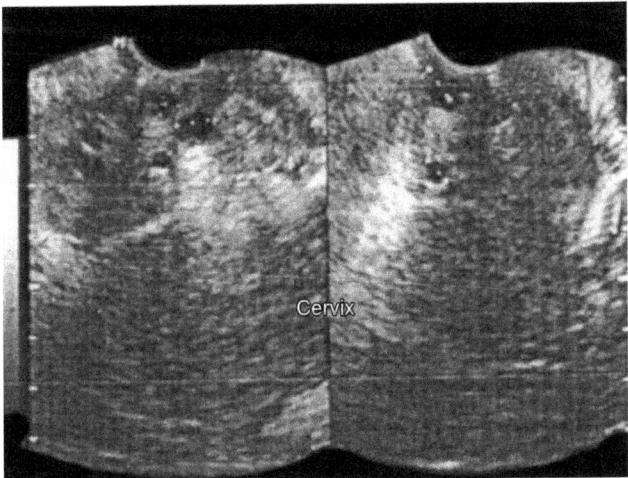

**Fig. 9.4:** Multiple ectatic endocervical glands (Nabothian cysts).

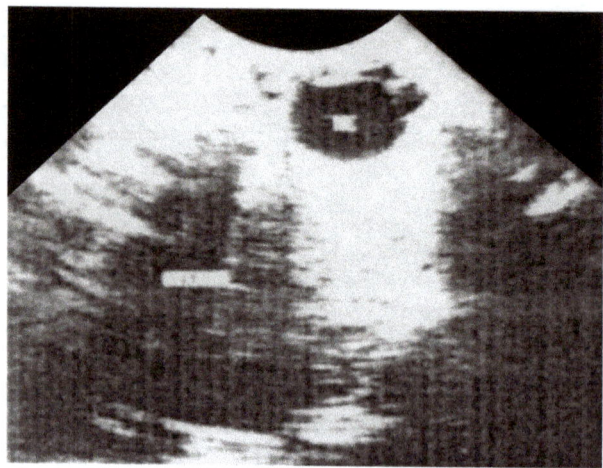

**Fig. 9.5:** Solitary nabothian cyst seen in the cervix.

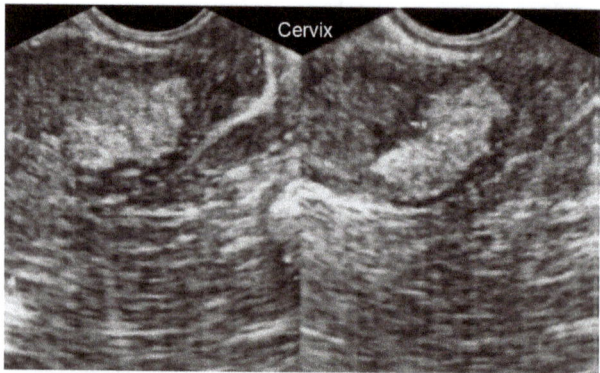

**Fig. 9.6:** Inhomogeneous ill-defined mass seen in the left wall of the cervix.

## Cervical Polyps

Arise from hyperplastic cervical epithelium due to chronic cervicitis, usually small <1 cm.

*On USG:* Appears as circumscribed, sessile, echogenic or hypoechoic. Color Doppler demonstrates a vascular pedicle. They are better appreciated during periovulatory period because better delineated by anechoic mucus.

## Cervical Stenosis

Occurs due to previous instrumentation like D&C, postmenopausal cervical atrophy, cervical carcinoma, radiation therapy, cone biopsy. Due to all reasons, fluid collection occurs within the uterine cavity.

*On USG:* Fluid as an anechoic area in endometrial cavity, fluid may contain internal echoes, debris, fluid filled level or gas.

## Cervical Pregnancy

In this embryo implanted in cervical mucosa distal to internal cervical os, account for less than 1% of all pregnancies.

*On USG:* Cervical pregnancy barrel shaped cervix containing gestation, with empty uterus with thick hyperechoic decidual reaction, with positive urine pregnancy test. No adnexal mass, otherwise normal pelvis are diagnostic criteria on USG.

## Cervical Carcinoma

Most common female genital carcinoma.

*On USG:* Demonstrate bulky large cervix, cervical width > 4 cm, anechoic fluid collection in uterine cavity due to cervical stenosis.

*On CD:* Abundant color flow in seen.

## Abnormal Vagina

The most common lesions visualized with sonography are (a) Gartner's duct cysts **(Figs. 9.7 and 9.8)**, (b) cryptomenorrhea.

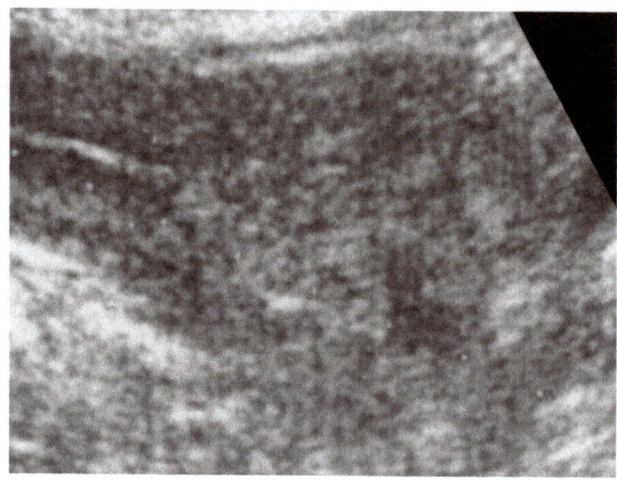

Cryptomenorrhea

**Fig. 9.7:** Inhomogeneous mass seen in the cervix.

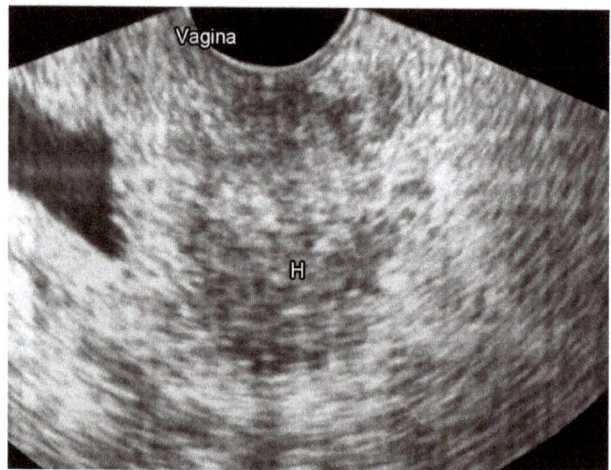

**Fig. 9.8:** Mass seen superior to the vaginal vault.

## Cryptomenorrhea

In this there is periodic shedding of endometrium and bleeding occurs but menstrual blood fails to come out from genital tract due to obstruction in the passage.

Causes congenital due to imperfect hymen, transverse vaginal septum, atresia of upper 1/3rd of vagina and cervix.

Acquired (1) Stenosis of cervix following amputation, conization, deep cauterization. (2) Secondary vaginal atresia following difficult/neglected vaginal delivery.

*On USG:* Vagina is seen with blood (hematocolpos), uterus is pushed upward and seen with blood filled (hematometra) → hematosalpinx (tubes filed with blood) seen.

## ABNORMALITIES OF FALLOPIAN TUBE (FIGS. 9.9 TO 9.11) ECTOPIC PREGNANCY

### Ectopic Pregnancy

Pregnancy that occurs outside the uterine cavity is called ectopic pregnancy. Most common site is fallopian tube 9 ff.

*Risk factors*: Pelvic inflammatory disease (PID), assisted reproductive technique (ART), previous tubal surgery, previous history of ectopic pregnancy, previous abortion, intrauterine contraceptive device (IUCD).

Transvaginal sonography (TVS) is of gold standard diagnostic modality for the effective and fast detection of ectopic pregnancy. The diagnostic signs of an ectopic pregnancy: (a) direct and (b) indirect.

*Direct signs*: Visualization of ectopic sac with or without a yolk sac and embryo.

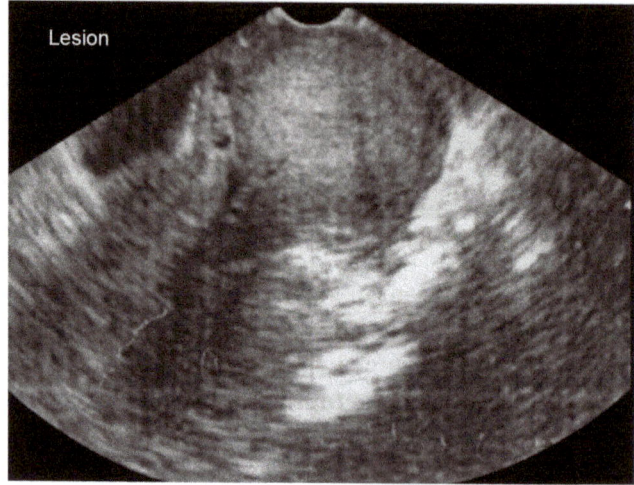

**Fig. 9.9:** Large mass seen in the vagina.

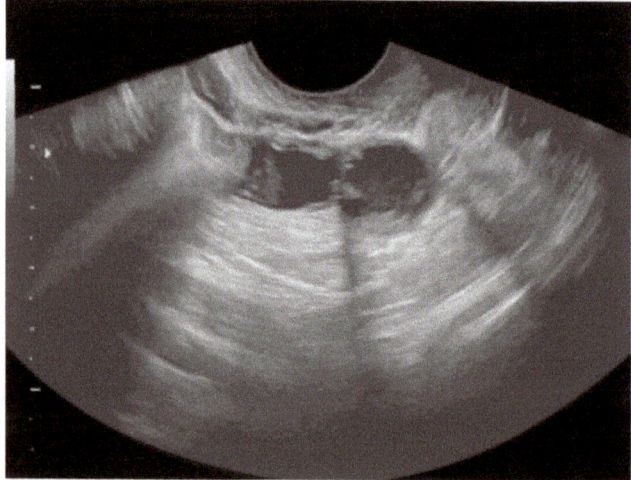

**Fig. 9.10:** Left hydrosalpinx with the left ovary seen separately.

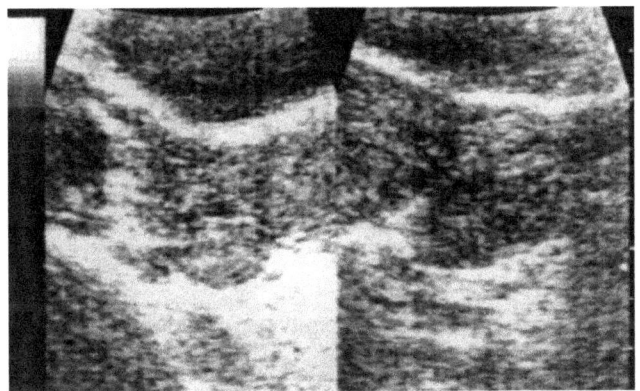

**Fig. 9.11:** Normal fallopian tubes as seen on ultrasound.

*Indirect signs*:

- Nonvisualization of an intrauterine sac (empty uterus) with HCG level greater than the discriminatory zone (1500-2000 iu/L).
- Pseudogestational sac inside the uterus.
- Complex, poorly defined, extraovarian adnexal mass.
- Tubal ring (echo fluid structure inside the tube).
- Abnormal tubal content (due to clots).
- Free fluid in POD, pelvis, abdomen.

*On CD:* Shows randomly dispersed multiple small vessels within the adnexa, show high velocity and low impedance signals (peripheral vascularization (ring of fire pattern) clearly separated from two ovarian tissues and corpus luteum.

## Acute Salpingitis

Inflammation of fallopian tubes (acute pelvic inflammatory disease).

On USG:
- Dilated tubular structure (retort-shaped), differentiated from pelvic vessels by using color Doppler and absence of pulsations, from bowel by absence of peristaltic movement.
- Echogenic thick tubal wall (thickness > 5 mm) which reflect inflamed mucosal lining.
- Cogwheel sign (sonolucent cogwheel-shaped structure with thick wall on cross section).
- Presence of incomplete septations.

Because of continuous spillage of inflamed material from the tube into surface of ovary, result in development of complex adnexal mass [tubo-ovarian (TO) complex].

*On USG:* In TO-complex, both tube and ovaries, identified clearly but cannot be separated from each other by pushing the tube with TVS probe.

With continuous disease, there is total breakdown of architecture of one or both adnexa, on USG neither the ovary nor the fallopian tubes are separately recognized and USG shows lobulated fluid collections in adnexal region and in cul de sac which is regarded as tubo-ovarian abscess. In which, features of marked tenderness at the touch of TVS probe are also seen.

*On CD:* Acute cases show high velocity blood flow RI = 0.53 ± 0.09 due to vasodilatation mediated by inflammation.

## Chronic Cases of Salpingitis

*USG features:*
- Distended tubes, thin-walled (<5 mm), with incomplete septae.
- Hyperechogenic knots (remnants of endosalpingeal folds) in cross section of fluid filled distal tissue shelter (Beads on-a-string sign).

*On CD:* Shows high resistance flow, i.e. RI 0.71 ± 0.09.

## Hydrosalpinx

When fimbrial or cornual end of tubes are closed, accumulation of mucus occurs in tubal lumen and this entity is called hydrosalpinx. Seen in cases of chronic PID.

*On USG:* Appears as a fusiform anechoic lesion in adnexal region.

*On 3D USG:* Shows sausage-shaped structure, it also helps to identify partial septations, caused by tubal folds, these two are important structures for differentiating cyst from hydrosalpinx.

## Fallopian Tube Carcinoma

Rarest of all gynecological malignancies Triad of pain, bleeding p/v, leucorrhea is pathognomonic of tubal carcinoma.

*On 2D USG:* Shows complex predominantly cystic adrenal mass or sausage shaped structure apparently separated from the uterus.

*On 3D TVS:* Enables clinician true perception, spatial relations 3D PD show futures of neovascularization with RI (0.38).

## Tubal Evaluation

Tubal occlusion is single most common cause of female infertility. Its evaluation is first step in an investigation of infertility.

Method by which done ultrasonographically called sonosalpingography: also known as Sion test. In this using saline as a contrast media, patency of tube is evaluated with help of TVS, by visualizing special fluid from fimbrial end of fallopian tube.

Normally fallopian tubes are isoechoic, and not visualized unless pathological or surrounded by fluid.

Patency is confirmed by free spillage of saline into peritoneal cavity.

On color Doppler spillage into peritoneal cavity shows waterfall sign (seen as bruit of color).

Prior to procedure, patient is asked to evacuate the bladder and no 8 Foleys catheter is put inside the uterus, Foleys balloon is inflated with 1–2 mL of distilled water. 20–60 mL solution containing ciplox, hyalase and dexamethasone are taken into a 20 mL syringe and pushed via Foleys catheter and spillage seen from fimbrial end. Then Foleys bulb is deflated and a small amount of saline is pushed slowly to evaluate the uterine cavity as sonohysterography.

When the SSG is done by using positive contrast media (e.g. echovist), the procedure is as HyCoSy (hysterocontrast-salpingography).

The SSG is good, noninvasive screening to evaluate the tubal patency.

## CUL-DE-SAC OR POUCH OF DOUGLAS

One can find fluid in the pouch of Douglas (POD) mostly in cases of infection **(Figs 9.12 to 9.17)**.

Space above the peritoneal recess comprising the posterior aspect of the uterus and anterior aspect of the rectum is called the POD. This is the most dependent part of female pelvis. Any free fluid of pelvis is first seen in this space.

Following structures can be in the POD:

*Bowel*: Identified by peristaltic movement.

*Fallopian tubes*: Seen floating in free fluid in POD. Stimulated ovaries during infertility fall in cul-de-sac behind the uterus.

Miscellaneous Disorders

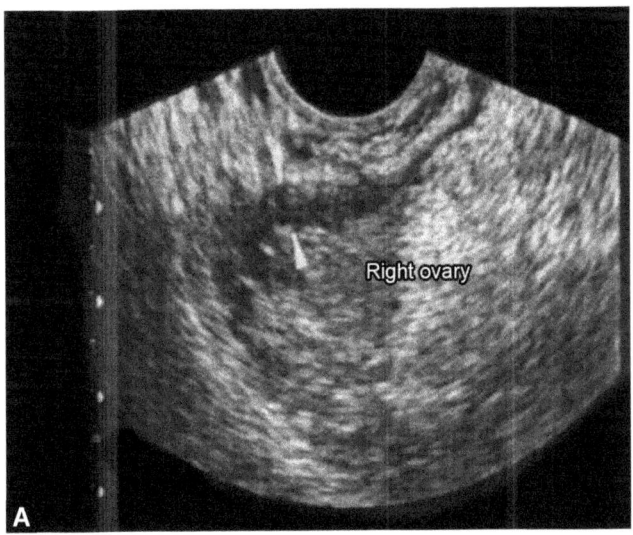

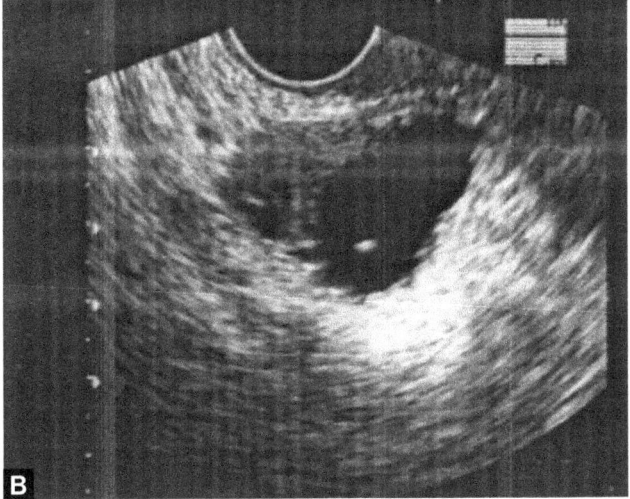

**Figs. 9.12A and B:** Ovary and hydrosalpinx seen in the right adnexa.

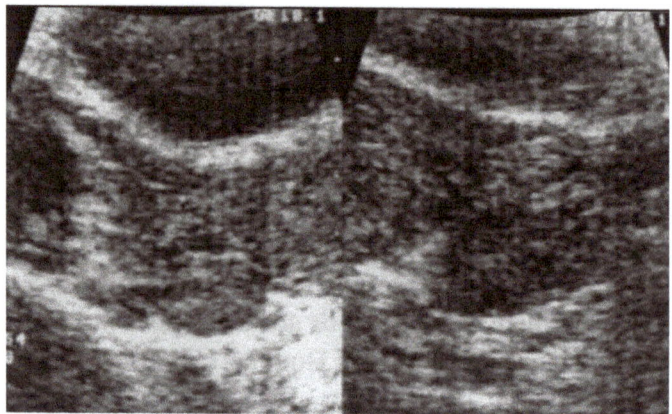

**Fig. 9.13:** Fluid in the pouch of Douglas seen in a case of acute pelvic inflammatory disease.

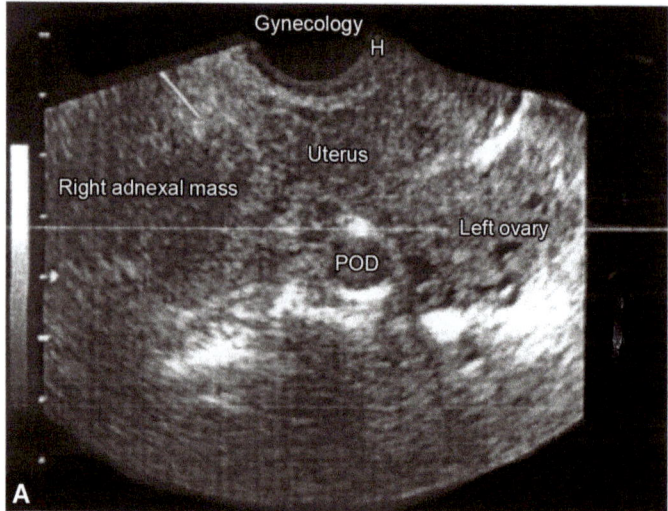

**Fig. 9.14A**

## Miscellaneous Disorders

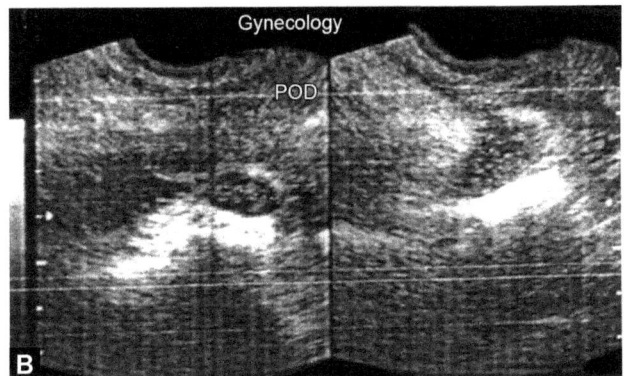

**Figs. 9.14A and B:** Fluid controls seen in the pouch of Douglas (POD).

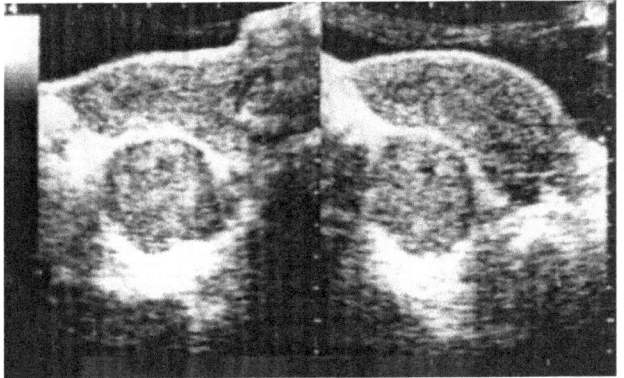

**Fig. 9.15:** Large hypoechoic fluid loculus seen in the pouch of Douglas.

*Peritoneal inclusion cysts*: Flimsy adhesions with fluid collection usually seen in patients after pelvic surgery or as a result of PID.

If large amount of free fluid in pelvis is seen, always look in hepatorenal pouch by TAS.

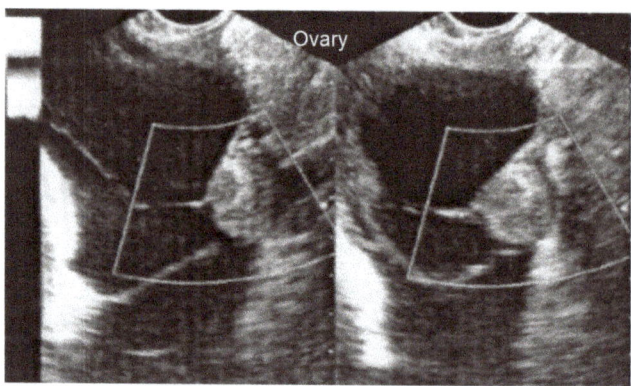

**Fig. 9.16:** Multiple loculi seen in the pouch of Douglas with the ovary seen lateral to it.

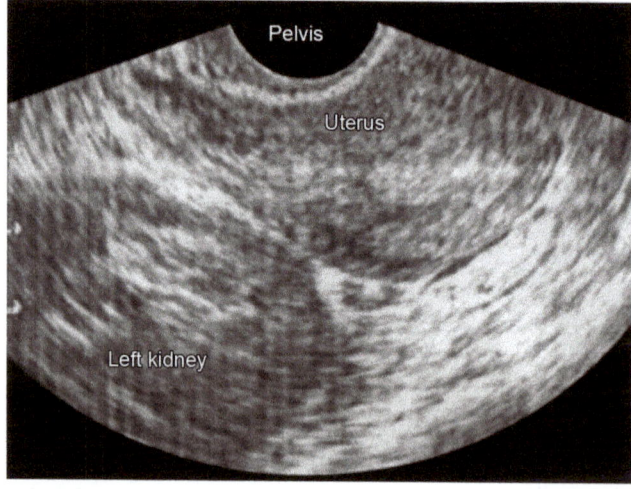

**Fig. 9.17:** Pelvic kidney seen initially as a mass in the pelvis.

# CHAPTER 10

# Ectopic Pregnancy

## INTRODUCTION

Ectopic pregnancy is the implantation of a fertilized ovum outside the uterine cavity. The successful treatment of tubal pregnancy with salpingectomy was first reported by Robert Lawson Tait in 1884.

## Incidence and Sites of Ectopic Implantation

The overall incidence of ectopic pregnancies is around 1 in 100 pregnancies.

## Presentation

Typical presentation is a triad of amenorrhea, abdominal pain, and irregular vaginal bleeding. Pain is usually located at either lower quadrant of the abdomen or lower back. Rupture of an ectopic pregnancy causes a sharp pain in the iliac fossa, followed by abdominal distension, generalized abdominal tenderness and guarding. The hemoperitoneum under the diaphragm cause referred pain to the shoulder. Massive intraperitoneal bleeding causes fainting or circulatory collapse. Vaginal bleeding in ectopic pregnancy is usually dark and scanty in amount.

| Type | Findings |
|---|---|
| Tubal | Tubal ring sign, ring of fire, pelvic hemorrhage |
| Interstitial | Eccentrically located gestational sac (G sac), interstitial line sign |
| Ovarian | β-HCG >1000, normal tubes, Gsac/adnexal mass in ovary or a typical cyst |
| Cervical | Trophoblastic flow surrounding Gsac within cervix, normal endometrium, ballooning of cervix, hourglass uterus |
| Scar pregnancy | Gsac within lower anterior segment of uterus, thinning of myometrium anterior to sac |
| Abdominal | Absence of IU Gsac, Gsac located within intraperitoneal cavity, pelvic hemorrhage |

The above table shows types of ectopic progress.

## Beta hCG

In normal pregnancy, serum concentration of beta hCG will increase exponentially in normal pregnancy, doubling every 2–3.5 days from the 4th to 8th weeks of gestation to reach a peak around 8th–12th weeks. Therefore, estimate of serum hCG at 48 hours interval is helpful.

If the increase of serum beta hCG is less than 85% or the level starts reaching a plateau or is decreasing, an ectopic pregnancy will be the most likely diagnosis.

## Ultrasound

- The ultrasonographic features of ectopic pregnancy are:
  - An empty uterus
  - An ectopic gestational sac or adnexal mass

- And/or varying amount of free fluid in pouch of Douglas and in the abdominal cavity.

Increased blood flow in the adnexal mass seen on Doppler ultrasound scan is suggestive of ectopic pregnancy.

## Correlation of Beta hCG Level and Ultrasound Examination

In normal intrauterine pregnancy, a gestational sac can be visualized in uterine cavity via transvaginal ultrasound as early as 5-week period of amenorrhea or serum beta hCG level of 1500 mIU/mL and via transabdominal ultrasound at 6-week period of a amenorrhea or serum beta hCG level of 3000 mIU/mL. The double ring or double decidual sign of gestational sac is the hallmark of intrauterine pregnancy, whereas single layer (pseudo sac) would be seen inside the uterus in ectopic pregnancy.

## Management of Ectopic Pregnancy

The treatment modalities available are:
- Expectant management
- Medical therapy with methotrexate
- Surgical intervention.

## Management of Ruptured Ectopic Management

- If the patient with ruptured tubal ectopic pregnancy is in shock or is unstable hemodynamically due to significant hemoperitoneum, laparotomy is the only rational approach in order to save her life.

- Salpingectomy or salpingostomy for affected tube depending on the state of contralateral fallopian tube.
- If the contralateral tube is damaged or absent congenitally, salpingostomy may be carried out to preserve the affected tube.
- Cornual resection will be the only procedure for *ruptured cornual pregnancy*. For women with torrential bleeding from *cervical ectopic pregnancy*, hysterectomy is the only option in order to save the woman's life.

## Surgical Management

- Laparoscopy is the preferred surgical approach in the hemodynamically stable patient with unruptured ectopic pregnancy. It appears to have a subsequent higher intrauterine pregnancy rate and lower recurrent ectopic pregnancy rate compared to laparotomy. Conservative method for tubal ectopic pregnancy is *salpingostomy*.
- *Salpingostomy* is usually procedure for tubal ectopic pregnancy. During this procedure, the part of the fallopians tube which contains ectopic gestational sac is removed by dissecting along the mesosalpinx and securing hemostasis.

Despite increase in the incidence of ectopic pregnancy, advances and availability of better u/s machines, transvaginal sonography (TVS) probes and expertise, have vastly improved the scenario of ectopic pregnancy. Not only fatal outcomes have tremendously decreased as compared to past but also owing to early diagnosis and intervention, the need for surgery has also decreased. Most of the times conservative management is successful, thus leaving scope for future fertility.

## Sonographic features of intrauterine and ectopic pregnancy

| Intrauterine pregnancy | Ectopic pregnancy | | |
|---|---|---|---|
| • Gestational sac of normal size and shape inside the uterine cavity | Uterine findings | Diagnostic signs | • Absence of gestational sac located in cavity<br>• Absence of embryo or its parts in the cavity |
| • Double ring<br>• Clear embryonic echo<br>• Positive heart action | | | |
| | Suggestive signs | | • Enlarged uterus<br>• Thick endometrium<br>• Free fluid in cul-de-sac |
| | Adnexal findings | | • Ectopic gestational sac with or without living embryo<br>Or<br>• Mixed solid and cystic mass |

The TVS has a sensitivity of 96% and specificity of 88%, combined with serum beta hCG, it is 100% and 99% respectively.

*Intrauterine findings are (Figs. 10.1A to D):*
- Empty uterus with or without increased endometrial thickness.
- Central sac like structure—the so called pseudogestational sac in 10-20%. Its shape changes with myometrial contractions. Color and pulsed Doppler are very useful here.

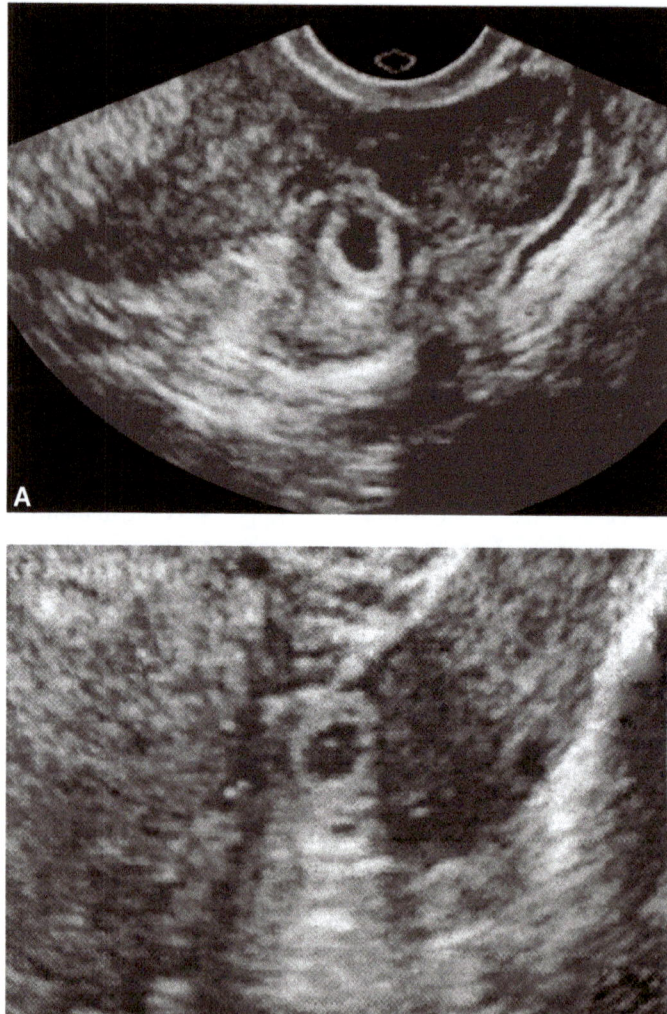

**Figs. 10.1A and B**

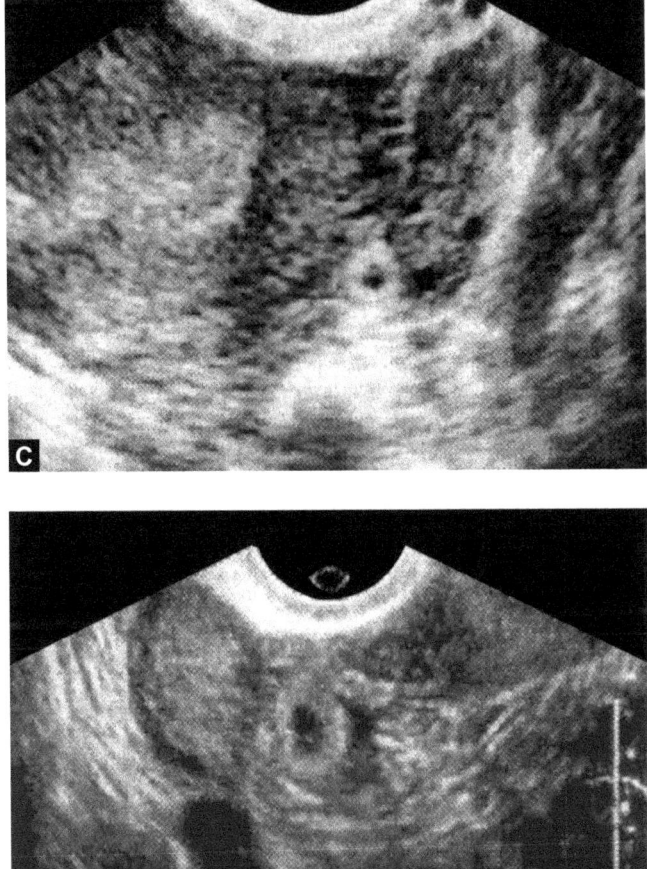

**Figs. 10.1A to D:** Transvaginal ultrasounds demonstrating ring-like structures situated between the uterus and ovary.

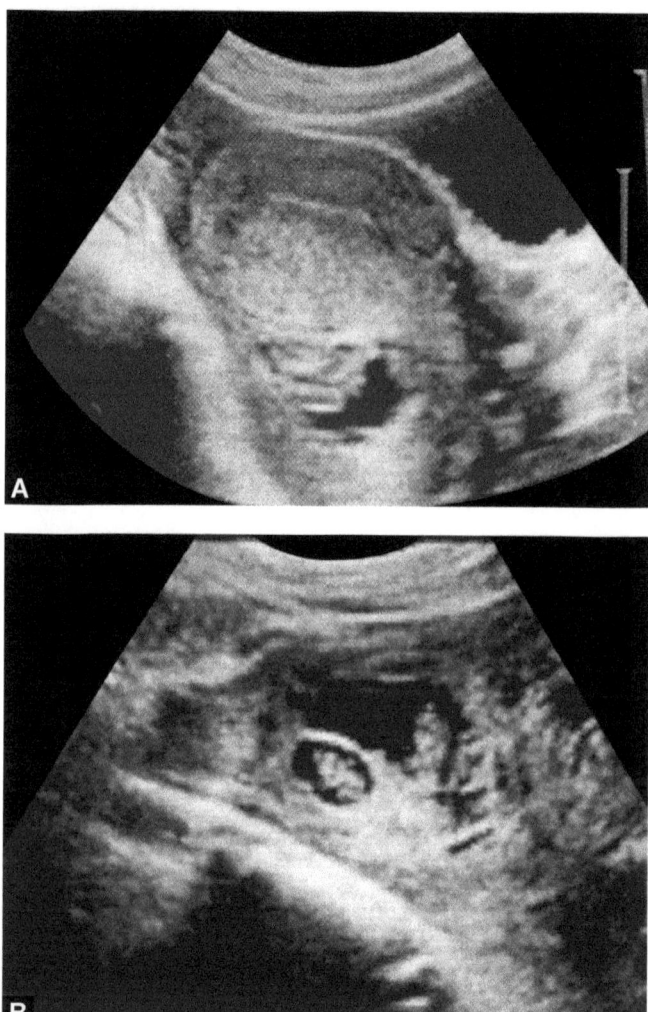

**Figs. 10.2A and B:** Transabdominal ultrasounds showing twin ectopic pregnancies.

*Adnexal findings are (**Figs. 10.2A and B**):*
- Gestational sac with clear embryonic echo and heart activity (15–28% only, viable ectopic).
- Gestational sac without heart activity.
- The commonest finding is an unspecific mass that moves away from ovary (blob sign).
- Empty gestational sac (bagel sign) in 20%.
- Presence of fluid in hepatorenal recess of subhepatic space.

Differential diagnosis on u/s
- Corpus luteum (CL)—eccentrically located within the ovary, surrounded by ovarian tissue. Echogenicity is slightly lower than that of ectopic. Hemorrhagic CL is hypoechoic rather than having a central cystic area **(Fig. 10.3)**.

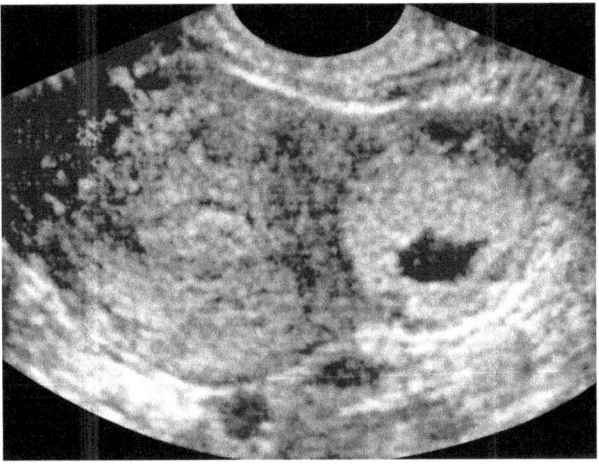

**Fig. 10.3:** The "ring of fire" pattern observed with the application of color Doppler does not distinguish between an ectopic pregnancy and an exophytic corpus luteal cyst. Separation of the mass and ovary occurred when transducer pressure was applied to the ovary, suggesting ectopic pregnancy. This was confirmed in the operating suite.

- Thick-walled ovarian follicle.
- Small intestine.
- Hydrosalpinx.
- Cystic adnexal masses like cystadenoma, cystadenofibroma, endometrioma, teratoma and pedunculated fibroids.
- In ART patients a large no. of artificial corpora lutea.

Free intraperitoneal fluid is seen in 40-83% of ectopic pregnancies but also in 20% of normal intrauterine pregnancies. Possibility of ectopic pregnancy increases if amount of fluid is moderate to large.

*Color flow pattern*—Randomly dispersed multiple small vessels within adnexa. **Figure 10.3** showing high velocity, low impedance signals (RI = 0.36-0.45) clearly separated from ovarian tissue and corpus luteum.

Luteal flow is detected on same side as the ectopic pregnancy.

*3D ultrasound* offers some advantage. Planar mode tomograms are helpful in distinguishing between true and pseudogestational sacs. 3D power Doppler may help in deciding conservative/active line of treatment.

*Other sites of implantation*
*Interstitial* (1.1-6.3%) **(Fig. 10.4)**
- Empty uterine cavity.
- Chorionic sac seen separately and more than 1 cm from most lateral edge of uterine cavity, surrounded by a thin myometrial layer.
- Approximately 15% of interstitial pregnancies may have heterotopic pregnancy. In such cases intrauterine findings may be misleading. Visualization of interstitial part of tube in close proximity of end and depiction of trophoblastic tissue is diagnostic.
- 3D ultrasound is very helpful in diagnosis.

*Cervical pregnancy* (incidence 1 in 50,000) **(Figs. 10.5 to 10.7)**

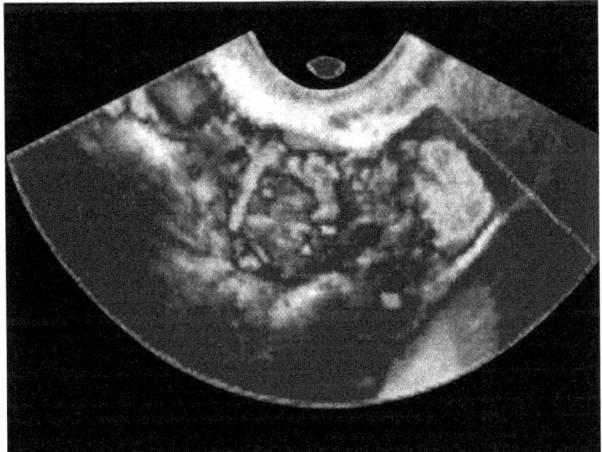

**Fig. 10.4:** Transvaginal ultrasound in a transverse plane showing an interstitial pregnancy.

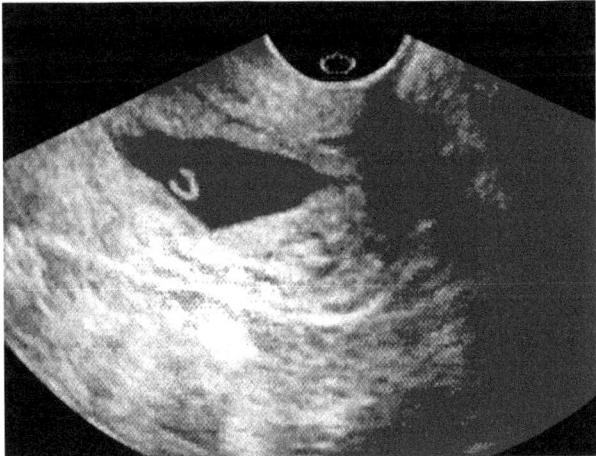

**Fig. 10.5:** Transvaginal ultrasound in long axis showing a gestational sac with yolk sac within the cervix.

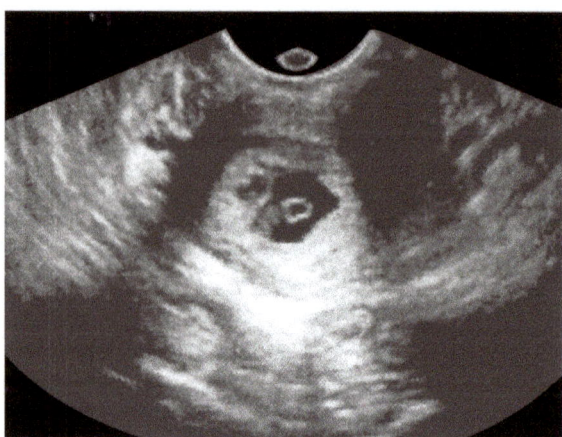

**Fig. 10.6:** Transvaginal ultrasound in a short axis view of the cervix showing a fetal pole within the gestational sac.

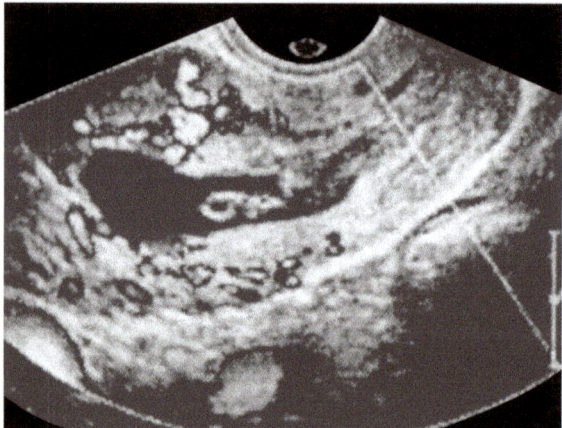

**Fig. 10.7:** Transvaginal ultrasound showing peritrophoblastic blood flow on color Doppler suggesting implantation of the gestational sac into the cervix.

- No evidence of intrauterine pregnancy
- An hour glass uterine shape with ballooned cervical canal
- Presence of gestational sac or placental tissue within cervical canal
- Closed internal os
- Color Doppler is very helpful in showing extensive vascular supply within cervix.
- 30 u/s is very helpful.

*Ovarian pregnancy (incidence less than 3% of ectopics):* Detection is by presence of hyperechoic trophoblastic ring within ovary. Color Doppler is very helpful by detection of peritrophoblastic flow.

*Intra-abdominal pregnancy (1% of all ectopic gestations):* The diagnosis of abdominal pregnancy is not easy especially in early stage.

*Pregnancy of unknown location (PUL):* Pregnancy of unknown location is the term used for a pregnancy with positive urine test but no pregnancy visualized on TVS. Specialized early pregnancy departments have estimated that between 8% and 10% of women attending for u/s will be classified to have PUL. The true nature of PUL can be:

- Ongoing viable intrauterine 30–47%
- Failed pregnancy 50–70%
- Ectopic pregnancy 6–20%
- Rarely a persisting PUL.

Persisting PUL is where hCG level does not spontaneously decline and no intrauterine or ectopic pregnancy is identified on follow-up TVS. A persisting PUL is likely to be either a small ectopic that has not been visualized, or a retained trophoblast in endometrial cavity.

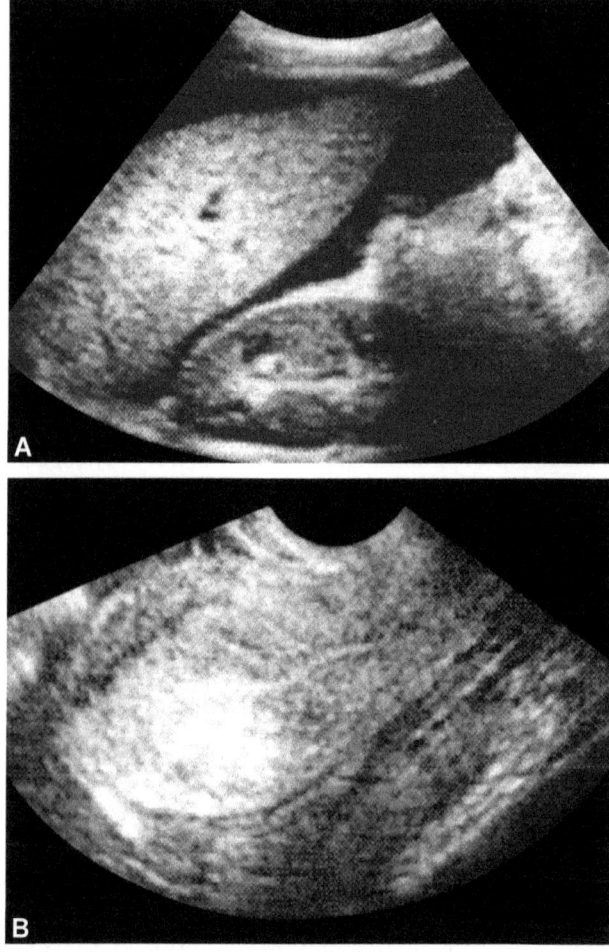

**Figs. 10.8A and B:** Transabdominal ultrasound showing a large amount of free fluid in and around the hepatorenal space in a patient with a ruptured ectopic pregnancy. Despite the amount of hemorrhage, free fluid was not readily seen on transvaginal ultrasound because of distorted landmarks from clotted blood (B).

## CONCLUSION

It is expected that increased sensitivity of the serum beta hCG immunoassay and the quality of transvaginal B-mode, color Doppler u/s and more recently 3D with color and power Doppler facilities will allow even earlier detection and conservative management of ectopic pregnancies **(Figs. 10.8A and B)**. Furthermore, it seems that fertility outcome and number of women attempting to conceive after ectopic pregnancy will further increase.

# CHAPTER 11

# Trophoblastic Disease in First-trimester

Outcome of trophoblastic disease has greatly improved by the introduction of ultrasound diagnosis early in pregnancy and management thereafter. Ultrasonically diagnosed early stage evacuation is easier than the later stage of developed molar mass. There can be total or partial molar pregnancy.

## TOTAL HYDATIDIFORM MOLE (FIGS. 11.1 AND 11.2)

Here chromosomes are usually diploid 46XX, where the XX are both of male origin that is called androgenesis. It is detected by TVS by the **(Tables 11. 1 and 11. 2)**:
- Presence of mole cysts in uterine cavity without fetus/embryo or its parts.
- Rarely an embryo with heart beat is detected earlier and approximately 4 weeks, later total mole may be found.
- Walls of empty gestational sac may show small cystic change before the typical growth of the total mole.
- Early total mole resembles a blighted ovum whereas vomiting and high hCG titers are contradictory. The gestational sac wall increases and typical molar cysts develop within 1–2 weeks.
- It is cystic but not snow storm pattern in modern B-mode device.

## Trophoblastic Disease in First-trimester

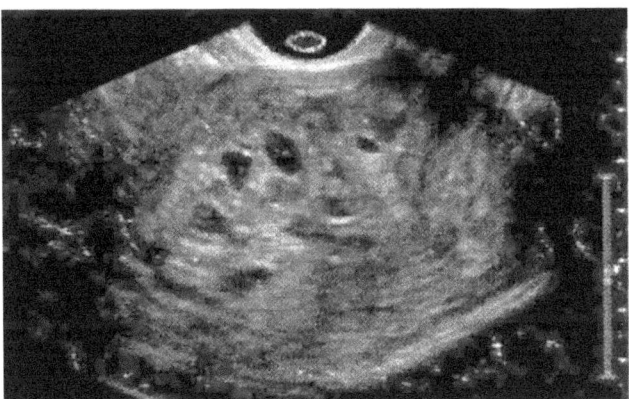

**Fig. 11.1:** Presence of molar cysts in uterine cavity.

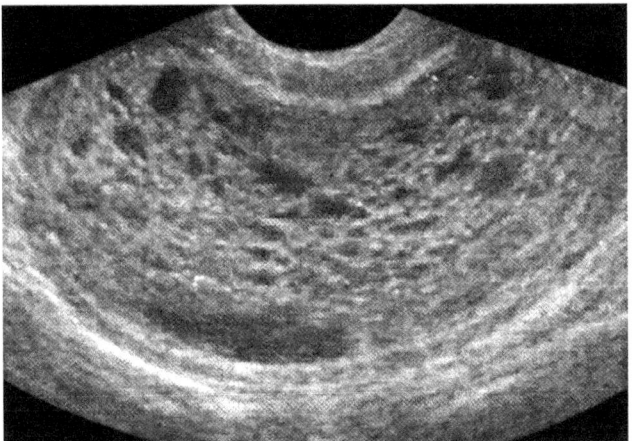

**Fig. 11.2:** Pelvic ultrasound of molar pregnancy

- On color Doppler diastolic flow is large and RI is lower in uterine, arcuate, radial and spiral arteries than normal pregnancy. RI is low in intervillous space also.

### Table 11.1: Symptoms of hydatidiform mole.

- Vaginal bleeding
- Passage of vesicles
- Anemia
- Hyperemesis gravidarum
- Pre-eclampsia
- Thyrotoxicosis
- Respiratory symptoms
    - Trophoblastic embolization
    - Thyroid storm

### Table 11.2: Signs of hydatidiform mole.

- Pallor
- Signs of pre-eclampsia
    - Elevated BP
    - Proteinuria
- Signs of hyperthyroidism
    - Tachycardia
    - Tremor
- Uterus larger than gestation
- Absence of fetal parts
    - External ballottement
    - Fetal heart sounds
- Doughy consistency
- Vaginal bleeding
- Ovarian cysts on pelvic examination

- Total hydatidiform mole develops in one of the twins or triplets also. In this case molar tissue is separated by the septum from the fetus.
- Total mole is diagnosed when urinary or serum hCG is higher than 100,000 µ/mL that is the higher normal range of early pregnancy **(Table 11.3)**.

**Table 11.3:** Diagnosis of hydatidiform mole.

- History
- Clinical examination
- Ultrasonography
    - Complex, echogenic intrauterine contents with cystic anechoic spaces called snow storm appearance
    - Absence of fetal parts
    - Absence of amniotic fluid
    - Theca lutein cysts
- β-hCG level
    - Higher than in normal pregnancy
- Determination of ploidy by flow cytometry
- Immunostaining for protein that is expressed by maternal gene

**Table 11.4:** Diagnosis of partial hydatidiform mole.

- Vaginal bleeding
- Uterus appropriate for gestational age
- No hyperemesis/pre-eclampsia/hyperthyroidism
- No theca lutein cysts **(Table 5)**
- Ultrasonography
    - Cystic spaces in the placenta
    - Reduced amniotic fluid
    - Fetus with growth retardation
    - Increased transverse diameter of the gestational sac
- Usually diagnosed on histopathology
- hCG elevation not marked
- Progression to GTN in 2–4%

# PARTIAL HYDATIDIFORM MOLE

- U/s shows the fetus or the partial image of fetus and partial changes of placental villi into molar cysts.
- Anomalies are common in the fetus **(Table 11. 4)**.

- Chromosomal examination shows triploidy 69XXX, 69XXY, or 69XYY. DNA analysis confirms androgenetic mechanism.

**Table 11.5:** Risk factors for development of gestational trophoblastic neoplasia.

- Uterus larger than gestation
- Pre-evacuation hCG > 100,000 μ/mL
- Theca lutein cysts > 6 cm in size
- Age > 40 years

# CHAPTER 12

# Intrauterine Contraceptive Device

## THE CLINICAL PROBLEM

Intrauterine contraceptive devices (IUDs), are a highly effective means of contraception with relatively few systemic side effects.

Modern IUDs that contain copper or slowly releasing levonorgestrel, over a number of years are now being used because infection is very rare with these devices. Usually inserted to prevent pregnancy, hormone-containing may also be used to prevent dysfunctional bleeding.

The proper location of an IUD, regardless of its type, is in the endometrial cavity at the fundus. The remainder of the device should be above the cervix. The nylon strings should be palpable or visible on pelvic examination. If this, cannot be identified, the, patient may referred for evaluation of a "lost IUD."

Some patients presenting for sonography have no other complaint other than a lost string. Others present with cramping, pain or abnormal bleeding. In either case the position of the IUD must be demonstrated. If the endometrium is empty, the device lies in the myometrium, has been expelled or has perforated the uterus. An IUD outside the uterus may not be seen on ultrasound because it is surrounded by gut.

When an IUD is in the correct location it always prevents a normal pregnancy but ectopic pregnancy may occur with copper-containing IUDs.

A pelvic sonogram may be requested before IUD insertion to ensure that there is no endometrial pathology, such as a submucosal myoma, or that the uterus is large to receive an IUD. Check sonogram are often performed after a difficult insertion with an oddly positioned uterus or after IUD removal to ensure that there is not much hemorrhage.

## TYPES OF DEVICES

### Copper-containing Devices

A number of earlier copper-containing IUDs were used in prior years, but today, only the Copper 380A, IUD is used. The IUD is a T-shaped device. Copper is wound around the base to prevent pregnancy. The shaft lies in the body of the uterus above the cervix in the endometrium with the wings (arms) lying transversely in the endometrium at the fundus extending toward the cornu. All portions of this IUD are densely echogenic and produce a shadow.

### Levonorgestrel-containing Devices

The Mirena IUD also has a T-shape and lies in a similar location. It is more difficult to see. The stem creates a shadow, but the echogenic source to the shadow is subtle; the proximal and distal ends of the shaft are echogenic. The arms are echogenic in a similar fashion to the copper 380A device. The Skyla IUCD is also T-shaped but is smaller and releases levonorgestrel over three years.

### IUDs in Use in Asia

Many different devices are used in other parts of the world, particularly in China. These vary in shape from circles to triangles.

## Older IUDs may Still be seen Occasionally

The Lippes Loop was the most widely used IUD, and there are still a few in use. In a long-axis view, the loop has two to five echogenic components, depending on whether a true long-axis IUD view has been obtained. Insertion of the Dalkon Shield was suspended some years ago because of a large number of associated infections, although it is possible some women still have it. The Dalkon Shield is the smallest of the IUDs. On both longitudinal and transverse scans, it appears as two echogenic foci. The Saf-T-Coil is an unusual older IUD that may still turn up. There are two spirals alongside a central stem.

## TECHNIQUE

### Intrauterine Device Position

*The transvaginal approach is essential.*
- If the IUD is in the uterus it will be seen no matter what is the uterine position, though a retroverted position may make visualization a little difficult. 3D views are better because they show the entire IUD including the arms, particularly in IUD's imbedded in the myometrium.
- The string is seen as a thin longitudinal echo, and if it is balled up then a small echogenic mass will be found near the inferior end of the IUD.
- If the IUD has perforated the myometrium, it often lies posterior to the uterus and can still be seen.
- If the IUD has perforated into the myometrium, the site and amount of intramyometrial extension are best seen by 3D.
- There are two echoes associated with an IUD known as "entrance" and "exit" echoes.

- Not all uteri are midline some may be oblique so scan accordingly.
- Presence of a submucosal myoma may displace an IUD into a different axis.
- The decidual reaction in the secretory phase may obscure an IUD, which can be appreciated by decreasing the gain.

## PATHOLOGY

### Lost IUD

*When the patient cannot feel the IUD strings in the vagina, it is termed as lost IUD.*

- In most of these cases the string is balled up and visible near the internal os.
- If an IUD is not seen on USG it may have expelled out or may have perforated the uterus and lying in the pelvis outside the uterus.
- If the IUD has perforated the myometrium, it often lies posterior to the uterus and can still be seen.

### Embedded IUDs

Some patients complain of pain and bleeding after IUD insertion. Bleeding is more common with copper-containing IUDs. An IUD which is located in the lower uterine segment and extending into the vagina or one which is too large for the uterine cavity may be painful or cause vaginal bleeding.

When the IUD is too low its arms get embedded in the myometrium because the shaft of the IUD is completely or partially in the cervix.

Copper-containing IUDs that are located below the fundal endometrial cavity are painful and ineffective.

Levonorgestrel-containing IUDs that are too low are often pain-free and may still prevent conception because they release levonorgestrel; a large series of patients with low or embedded Mirena IUCDs were reported to be without pain, and apparently the devices continued to function well.

The IUD may be too wide for the endometrial cavity. The standard IUD is 32 mm wide; in women with smaller uteri, the wings may extend into the cornu beyond the endometrial cavity. This can be uncomfortable. The smaller Skyla IUD has been developed for women with a thinner endometrium (less than 32 mm) on transverse C-scan views.

## Pregnancy

Pregnancy can occasionally occur with copper-containing IUDs. This complication is almost unknown with IUDs that contain levonorgestrel. When an IUD with a coexisting pregnancy is discovered, one should determine the relationship of the device to the gestational sac (i.e. superior or inferior). This relationship is important in deciding whether an IUD can be safely removed. If it is left in place, infection may occur, or the fetus may be damaged by contact with the IUD. In the later stages of pregnancy, the location of the IUD is difficult to determine because of the large volume of the uterus occupied by the fetus.

## Infection

IUDs have been historically associated with a slightly increased incidence of PID. If a patient presents with pain or bleeding and the IUD is properly positioned, check the adnexal areas and the cul-de-sac for evidence of PID. Thickening of the endometrium alongside the shaft may indicate endometritis or additional pathology within the endometrium, like a polyp.

## PITFALLS

- Do not mistake the shadow of the IUD for the true position of the IUD.
- When the patient is in the secretory phase of the cycle and the endometrium is thick, it may be difficult to see the IUD.
- The balled-up string in the region of the internal os may not be obvious.
- Magnify the image, and use 3D to see the subtle string components.
- Myomas may distort the endometrium, so that the IUD appears to lie off-axis.

### Lost IUD

- The IUD has been pulled/fallen out.
- The string is balled up in the cervix above the external os.
- The IUD is in the myometrium.
- The IUD is in the cul-de-sac.
- The IUD is in the bladder.

# CHAPTER 13

# Vaginal Bleeding with Negative Pregnancy Test

Vaginal bleeding between periods or at any time in the premenstrual or postmenstrual nonpregnant patient is abnormal and is an indication for a sonogram. Very heavy painful periods may indicate an endometrial process.

In a child, vaginal bleeding may be a sign of precocious puberty. Other clinical features that occur in the child with precocious puberty include large breasts (gynecomastia), excessive growth, and the development of an adult pubic hair distribution.

There are many possible reasons for menstrual bleeding. Conditions that cause abnormal bleeding but do not distort the normal pelvic anatomy (e.g. problems) cannot be detected by sonography.

Sonographically visible findings include the following:
- Retained products of conception.
- Fibroids that border on the endometrial cavity, especially submucosal intracavitary ones.
- Intracavitary masses, such as polyps, form a well-defined focal mass, whereas others, such as cancer of the endometrium or endometrial hyperplasia, cause an increased thickness or focal irregularity to the endometrial cavity borders.

- Adnexal masses—Occasionally, an ovarian mass, such as a hormone-secreting ovarian neoplasm or dermoid, may cause vaginal spotting.

## CHANGES WITH MENSTRUATION

The lining of the endometrial cavity is partially shed each month at menstruation, with consequent changes in cavity appearance during the course of the cycle. During the preovulatory (proliferative) phase, the endometrial cavity echo is only approximately 3 mm thick and surrounded by an echopenic halo. Shortly before ovulation, two additional linear echoes outline the echopenic area (the "three-line sign" or trilaminar appearance). The echopenic area becomes more echogenic so that in the postovulatory (secretory or luteal) phase, the cavity echo becomes brighter and thicker. At this point, the width of the canal is between approximately 8 and 13 mm.

Ascertain the following before starting a study for vaginal bleeding:
- Complete menstrual history—last menstrual period (LMP), regularity of cycle, duration of bleeding and amount of bleeding.
- How long ago did the patient stop menstruating, if menopausal?
- If the patient is postmenopausal, is she on hormone replacement therapy (HRT)? HRT with estrogen or a combination of estrogen and progesterone thickens the endometrium. Unopposed estrogen (estrogen only) is particularly likely to thicken the endometrium. A postmenopausal endometrial cavity thickness of greater than 5 mm in an unstimulated patient may require further investigation, such as a saline infusion study (SIS) or endometrial sampling.

- Is tamoxifen being administered? Tamoxifen, a commonly administered antiestrogenic chemotherapeutic drug, is given to women who have had breast cancer. Although it reduces breast cancer recurrence, there is a slight increase in the number of endometrial neoplasms. After six months to one year, 60% of women develop secondary changes in the endometrium.

## TECHNIQUE

### Transvaginal

The endometrium can only be satisfactorily assessed with the vaginal probe. Detail is never satisfactory with the transabdominal approach.

### Saline Infusion Study (Hysterosonogram)

- This technique is used for the further investigation of the cause of abnormal vaginal bleeding.
- Informed consent is usually obtained because the procedure involves placing a catheter within the endometrial cavity, although the risks of infection and bleeding are minimal.
- In patients with a history of pelvic inflammatory disease, antibiotic prophylaxis with an antibiotic such as doxycycline is given.
- Pain and cramping may occur if a balloon catheter is inserted; if that is planned, an analgesic such as ibuprofen is given before the procedure.
- The procedure is performed as follows:
  - A speculum is inserted.
  - The cervix is cleansed with an antiseptic.
  - A small catheter, such as a 5F Tampa catheter, is inserted into the cervix using sponge forceps. If

fibroids are present or the catheter will not stay in place, a 5F to 7F balloon catheter is inserted. The balloon is inflated with a fluid such as normal saline to prevent air within the balloon from causing a shadow that would make visualization of uterine pathology impossible. If the balloon is difficult to insert, a technique whereby the balloon is inflated, deflated, withdrawn, pushed in again, and then reinflated may be helpful in getting the catheter in place. A tapered plastic os dilator also helps ease the passage of the catheter in some cases.

## PATHOLOGY

### Endometrial Cancer

Endometrial cancer is most common after menopause and is associated with abnormal bleeding. Typically, there is an echogenic mass with a large (sessile) base arising from the endometrium. These cancers are highly vascular with many supplying vessels. The management is changed and prognosis is worse if the tumor penetrates the echopenic area around the endometrium in the myometrium. Fluid in the endometrial cavity may occasionally be an indication of an underlying endometrial neoplasm.

### Benign Endometrial Hyperplasia

The endometrium becomes thickened (greater than 8 mm thick) and echogenic in the first half of the cycle, the proliferative phase, when it is normally thin. The condition can either be generalized or localized to a small segment of the endometrium.

Small cysts may lie within the echo area in the cavity border. This condition usually seen around the time of menopause.

## Endometrial Polyp

Polyps within the endometrial cavity are common. Typically, they are round echogenic, have an irregular border, and can be seen to move if they are on a stalk, as they often are color flow shows a single supplying vessel to polyp about half the time. This finding favors a benign origin to the polyp. Almost no polyps are malignant. Polyps may be multiple and may be located anywhere in the endometrium or cervical canal. If the examination is performed in the secretory phase of the menstrual cycle, polyps may be concealed within normal echogenic thickening that at this phase of the cycle. Many are asymptomatic, but some present with heavy periods or intermenstrual bleeding. If there is, uncertainty whether a polyp is present a hysterosonogram is helpful. When outlined by fluid with a hysterosonogram.

## Fibroids

Fibroids that abut the endometrial (submucosal) or that lie within the endometrial cavity (intracavitary) are a frequent cause of heavy periods, intermenstrual spotting or occasionally postmenopausal bleeding. When outlined by fluid, during the performance of an SIS, they have a smooth, mildly echogenic border and less echogenic internal contents. They are immobile and can usually be seen to extend beyond the confines of the endometrial cavity.

## Retained Products of Conception

The cause of vaginal bleeding is seen in a woman who has been recently pregnant, has undergone an elective termination of pregnancy, or had a vaginal delivery. Transvaginal probe views will show echogenic material within the endometrial cavity, occasionally with an area of acoustic shadowing related to a bony fragment. As a rule, the retained product is a portion of the placenta and will have typical placental texture.

Blood and retained products can look very similar. An SIS can help differentiate blood from retained products because retained products will adhere to the endometrium, whereas blood will float around. Color flow Doppler is also helpful because retained placenta that is attached to the uterine wall often shows blood perfusion when examined with color flow; blood clot never lights up with color flow.

If the endometrial cavity appears empty, this is helpful to the referring clinician because it means that there are no significant retained products.

## Recurrence of Apparent Menstruation after an Interval of Months or Years

Menopause does not occur abruptly. A genuine period with ovulation may occur after a gap of months or years. In a patient with recurrent menstruation after a long gap (e.g. two years), the endometrium may be thick if the patient is in the secretory phase or a cyst representing a follicle will be seen in an ovary.

## Atrophic Endometrium

After the patient is menopausal, providing she is not taking HRT, the endometrium normally measures 4 mm or less. This atrophic endometrium can bleed spontaneously because it is fragile. Providing the outline of the endometrium is smooth without a focal mass and no blood dyscrasias is present, one can presume that postmenopausal bleeding relates to an atrophic endometrium. This is important because the patient does not need a biopsy or other invasive intervention.

## Postmenopausal Hormone Replacement Therapy

HRT prevents postmenopausal side effects such as hot flashes and helps to prevent osteoporosis, so it is still used by some patients. Most women take sequential estrogen and progesterone, which mimics the premenopausal appearance. In women who take estrogen alone, the endometrium can look very thick because this regimen promotes endometrial hyperplasia. Much smaller continuous doses of estrogen coupled with progesterone give a mildly thickened endometrium and is useful preventing postmenopausal symptom, such as hot flashes.

## Cesarean Section Scar

Women who have had a caesarean section performed are left with a scar. The pouch related to the scar may fill with blood at the time of menstruation; old dark blood leaks out slowly over the next few days causing intermenstrual spotting. A giving caesarean section scar at the junction of the cervix and body of the uterus will be readily seen with the transvaginal probe.

## Tamoxifen

Tamoxifen changes are of two types:
1. Subendometrial cystic changes.
2. Multiple polyps.

## Ablation Breakdown

Ablation of the endometrium by different techniques is a common method of treating endometrial hyperplasia or AUB. At times this procedure fails in a portion and sonogram shows fluid/blood in the upper portion of the endometrium, which is painful as it passes through the cervical canal.

## Adenomyosis

It is a common cause of painful heavy periods.

## Polycystic Ovary Syndrome

Polycystic ovary syndrome, may be responsible for heavy or light periods and intermenstrual spotting.

## PITFALLS

- Intracavitary masses in the secretory phase of the cycle. The endometrial cavity echoes vary between 0.2 and 0.5 cm thick in the proliferative phase of the cycle and between 0.8 and 1.3 cm thick in the secretory phase of the cycle. Small masses such as polyps or intracavitary fibroids may be concealed in the secretory phase. If possible, schedule patients with possible intracavitary masses for the proliferative phase of the cycle or repeat the study.
- Blood clot versus intracavitary mass. In a patient with a history of intermenstrual bleeding or heavy periods, an apparent intracavitary mass may represent a blood clot. Blood clots usually move within the cavity when an SIS is performed. Blood clot is also seen if the patient is examined when she is menstruating.

# Vaginal Bleeding with Negative Pregnancy Test

- Transvaginal scanning with a bladder containing some urine. If the bladder is not completely empty reverberation artifacts may obscure crucial structures, and problem areas may be pushed far away from the transducer.
- SIS in the secretory phase. If a hysterosonogram is performed in the secretory phase, the endometrium is fragile. The catheter can push up the endometrium so it looks like a polyp. A polyp can be suspected when none is present because the borders of the cavity are often irregular in the secretory phase.
- Bubbles on a saline infusion study. Air can accumulate at the fundus and conceal pathology if the uterus is anteverted.

## DIFFERENTIAL DIAGNOSIS

- Submucosal or intracavity myoma/polyp
- Endometrial hyperplasia
- Atrophy (in postmenopausal patient)
- Adenomyosis
- Retained products (in post-pregnant patients)
  - IUDs
  - Recurrence of menstruation after apparent menopause
  - Post-endometrial ablation with partial endometrial breakdown
  - Hormone replacement therapy
  - Polycystic ovary syndrome.

# CHAPTER 14

# Chronic Pelvic Pain

## CLINICAL PROBLEM

- Chronic pelvic pain is common and responsible for approximately 10% of gynecological outpatient visits **(Table 14.1)**.
- Two common causes are endometriosis and the long-term consequence of pelvic inflammatory disease (PID).
- Typical symptoms are dyspareunia and dysmenorrhea, but muscular trigger pain, cannot be recognized with ultrasound.

**Table 14.1:** Chronic pelvic pain.

- Nature
  - Noncyclic pain
- Duration
  - 6 months or more
- Location
  - Lower abdomen
  - Low back
  - Buttocks
- Prevalence
  - 15–20%
- Age group
  - Reproductive age group

# TECHNIQUE (FLOWCHART 14.1)

## Tenderness

The transvaginal probe is superior to an examining finger because one can find the site of pelvic pain while pushing with the probe to see where the pain originates.

- Introduce the vaginal probe with care in symptomatic patients so as not to cause vaginal spasm and lack of cooperation in finding the cause of the pain. An alternative technique is to have the patient insert the vaginal probe in the vagina herself.
- Carefully push with a consistent pressure on the pelvic structures, including the proximal fallopian tubes, asking the patient to grade the severity of the pain from 1 to 10. (A score of 10 is the worst). Repeat the procedure several

**Flow chart 14.1:** Algorithm for evaluation and management of chronic pelvic pain.

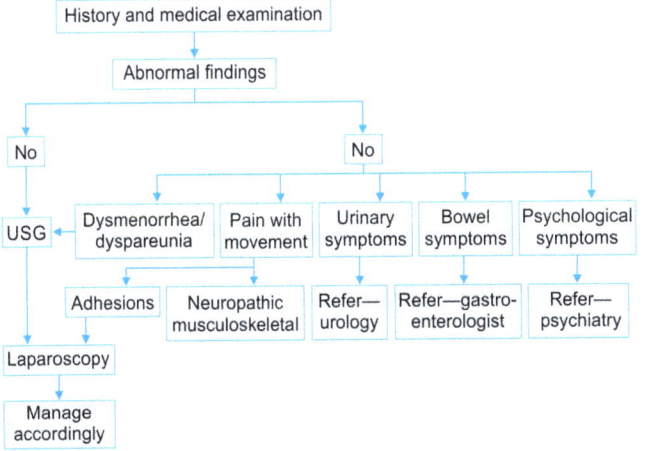

times if it is unclear where the pain is most severe so you can be sure where the pain originates. However, if it is obvious where the patient is maximally tender, you do not need to repeat this painful test. Do not be unnecessarily cruel; the test only works with patient cooperation.
- If the tenderness is superior to the area that can be examined with vaginal probe, feel the abdomen for the most painful site and look with the abdominal probe.

## Movement

Make sure that the uterus and ovaries move freely and slide away from neighboring structures such as the uterus, bowel, or side wall structures. Normally, the ovary can be pushed away from neighboring gut or the uterus if it lies adjacent to the uterus, and the uterus will slide away from the gut posterior to it as it is depressed. Convincing absence of free movement indicates adhesions.

## PATHOLOGY

## Chronic Pelvic Inflammatory Disease (Table 14.2)

- Chronic pain related to an earlier infection with PID is common and usually unrecognized unless the sonographer accurately localizes the tenderness. In this situation, tenderness is maximal over the proximal fallopian tubes and to a lesser extent over the uterus.
- Often, cultures are negative, and the only way to confirm that the right diagnosis has been made is that the pain disappears after the administration of a course of an antibiotic such as doxycycline.

> **Table 14.2:** Causes of chronic pelvic pain.

- Gynecological conditions
  - Endometriosis
  - Chronic PID
  - Pelvic adhesions
  - Adenomyosis
  - Ovarian remnant/residual ovary syndrome
  - Pelvic congestion syndrome
  - Leiomyoma
- Urological conditions
  - Interstitial cystitis
  - Urethral syndrome
  - Chronic urinary tract infection (UTI)
- Gastrointestinal conditions
  - Irritable bowel syndrome
  - Inflammatory bowel disease
- Musculoskeletal disorders
  - Separation of pubic symphysis
  - Sacroiliitis
  - Myofascial pelvic pain syndrome
- Neurological conditions
  - Nerve entrapment
  - Neuropathic pain
- Psychosomatic disorders
  - Anxiety
  - Depression
  - Sexual dysfunction

- Sometimes the pain relates to a hydrosalpinx. There is a serpiginous or apparently septate extraovarian mass. The walls of the dilated tube are thin, but there are intermittent small nodules representing the remnants of endosalpingeal folds.
- Hydrosalpinges may cause pain by distending to a point where they compress other organs. Usually they are

bilateral, but they may be of very different size on the two sides.
- The fallopian tubes may be enlarged and thickened due to chronic inflammation.
- They will be locally tender.

## Masses

Large, slowly growing uterine or adnexal masses may cause pain by compression of neighboring organs. Adenomyosis causes an enlarged tender uterus, dyspareunia, and dysmenorrhea.

## Infertility

Endometriosis is a common cause of pelvic pain that often causes infertility (**Table 14.3**). Often, the typical masses seen

| Table 14.3: Gynecological causes of chronic pelvic pain. | |
|---|---|
| *Condition* | *Associated features* |
| Endometriosis | • Dysmenorrhea<br>• Dyspareunia |
| Pelvic inflammatory disease (PID) | • History of STD/acute PID/IUCD<br>• Dysmenorrhea<br>• Dyspareunia |
| Adhesions | • History of prior surgery/PID/endometriosis<br>• Pain on movement |
| Adenomyosis | • Heavy menstrual bleeding<br>• Dysmenorrhea |
| Ovary remnant/trapped ovary syndrome | • History of hysterectomy<br>• Cyclic exacerbation of pain |
| Pelvic congestion syndrome | • Dyspareunia<br>• Pain on standing |

with endometriosis are absent, and the condition can only be inferred by the presence of adhesions. Unusual sites of endometriotic implants should be sought, such as incisions on the abdominal wall, bowel, and bladder wall.

## Adhesions

- Occur as a consequence of previous infection or surgery (e.g. tubal ligation)
- May be seen with endometriosis
- Occur occasionally with malignancy.

Adhesions may cause a chronic, nagging pelvic pain. Although the adhesions cannot be seen with ultrasound unless ascites is present, there are several indirect signs **(Tables 14.4 and 14.5)**:

- Uterine deviation to left or right or extreme retroversion.
- An ovary positioned in a high or low lateral position.

| Table 14.4: Urological causes of chronic pelvic pain. | |
|---|---|
| *Condition* | *Associated features* |
| Interstitial cystitis | • Dysuria<br>• Frequency<br>• Pain on bladder filling<br>• Allergens<br>• Irritable bowel syndrome |
| Urethral syndrome | • Dysuria<br>• Frequency<br>• Incontinence<br>• Post void fullness |
| Chronic/recurrent UTI | • Dysuria<br>• Frequency<br>• Systemic symptoms |

**Table 14.5:** Gastrointestinal/musculoskeletal/neurological causes of chronic pelvic pain.

| Condition | Associated features |
|---|---|
| • Gastrointestinal<br>   ▪ Irritable bowel syndrome<br>   ▪ Inflammatory bowel disease | • Altered stool frequency/consistency<br>• Altered stool passage<br>• Bloating<br>• Passage of mucus<br>• Bloody diarrhea |
| • Musculoskeletal conditions | • Pain on movement<br>• Worsen by end of day<br>• Trigger points |
| • Neurological conditions | • Location depends on the nerve involved<br>• Bladder/bowel/sexual dysfunction |

- An ovary located adjacent to the uterus that cannot be moved with the vaginal probe and is locally tender. This is a very reliable sign.
- An ovary that feels stiff and immobile when pushed with the transducer and that remains adjacent to a loop of bowel. Normally, the ovary can be pushed away from surrounding bowel with the transducer.
- A stiff feel as the vaginal probe is inserted indicates adhesions. As one performs more transvaginal sonograms, this sensation becomes more recognizable.

## Ovarian Remnant Syndrome

Sometimes, a remnant of one ovary remains after hysterectomy and bilateral salpingo-oophorectomy (surgical removal of the uterus and both ovaries). The ovarian remnant, produces follicles and corpora lutea, because it is surrounded by adhesions in a confined space, cyst formation is painful and occurs at approximately monthly intervals when ovulation takes place. Make sure that the patient is examined when she is symptomatic; you will be able to see the follicles or corpus luteum. Pushing on the mass will be very painful.

## Deep Pelvic Endometriosis

Endometrioma that develop deep in the pelvis in the cul-de-sac are notoriously difficult to diagnose and cause severe chronic pelvic pain. An echopenic mass develops the cul-de-sac often surrounding the urethra; local tenderness and mobility is characteristic of this syndrome.

## Pelvic Congestion Syndrome

Dilated veins in the region of the ovary particularly on the left, are found often and may occasionally be the cause of chronic pain. It is difficult to know when such varicosities are a genuine cause of symptoms and when they are coincidental. Approximately 10% of women have visibly dilated left pelvic veins, but a small minority have symptoms. Local vein tenderness when compressed with the vaginal probe maybe of some help in deciding if the veins any significance. Use color flow to establish that large cystic structures in the region of the ovary are dilated veins.

## Diverticular Disease

Painful diverticula in the sigmoid colon, which lies close to the left ovary, are often mistaken for a gynecologic process.

Diverticula are common, occurring in one-third of women aged more than 45 years. The bowel wall is abnormally thickened (greater than 2 mm) with a dome-shaped hump if a diverticular abscess is present. Small echogenic lines in the bowel wall suggest the presence of diverticula. Some contain shadowing gas. The bowel wall will be locally tender as it is pressed with the vaginal probe.

## Irritable Colon

This common condition leads to chronically thickened sigmoid bowel wall (greater than 2 mm thick), presumably due to focal spasm. Vaginal pressure on the thickened bowel wall reproduces the patient's symptoms **(Tables 14.6 to 14.8)**.

## Interstitial Cystitis

Bladder wall inflammation is often mistaken for a gynecologic lesion. In this condition, the wall of the bladder is exquisitely tender, and the bladder capacity is usually small (less than l00 mL). (To crudely calculate bladder volume in milliliters, measure the width, length, and height of the bladder and multiply by 0.65).

## PITFALLS

- If the patient has intermittent pain, make sure she is examined when she is having pain.
- Some patients gain sympathy from talking about pelvic pain. If the pressure test yields inconsistent results with the site of pain varying, make sure to report this.
- Tests for adhesions are often indeterminate. Make sure the ovary will not: move and is recognizably an ovary before

## Table 14.6: History in chronic pelvic pain.

- Location of pain (pain diagram)
- Precipitating factor
  - Posture
  - Prolonged standing
  - End of day
  - Coitus
- Type of pain
- Distribution
  - Lower abdomen
  - Low back
  - Thigh
  - Pelvic
- Intensity
- Associated symptoms
  - Dyspareunia
  - Dysmenorrhea
  - Frequency/dysuria
  - Bowel symptoms
- History of gynecological disorders
  - Endometriosis
  - Pelvic inflammatory disease
  - Tuberculosis
- History of surgery
  - Hysterectomy
  - Oophorectomy
  - Other surgeries
- History of psychiatric disorders
  - Social history
  - Sexual abuse
- History of medications

making this observation. The uterus is often deviated to the right or left or retroverted without adhesions being present.

**Table 14.7:** Physical examination in chronic pelvic pain.

- General examination
- Abdominal examination
  - Abdominal/pelvic mass
  - Trigger points
- Per speculum examination
  - Vaginal discharge
- Pelvic examination
  - Pelvic mass
  - Adnexal/uterine tenderness
  - Trigger points
- Per rectal examination
  - Uterosacral ligaments
- Examination of lumbar spine/sacroiliac joints

**Table 14.8:** Investigations in chronic pelvic pain.

- Complete blood count
- Venereal disease research laboratory (VDRL)
- Urinalysis and midstream culture
- Vaginal swab for culture/chlamydia
- Abdominal and transvaginal USG
  - Endometriosis
  - Tubo-ovarian mass
  - Adenomyosis
  - Residual/remnant ovary
- Urological and GI evaluation
- Laparoscopy
  - Endometriosis
  - Pelvic congestion syndrome
  - Adhesions
  - Pelvic inflammatory disease (PID)
- MRI and CT scan
  - Cardiorespiratory

# CHAPTER 15

# Common Gynecological Diseases

- Abnormalities due to presence or absence of androgens and antimüllerian hormone.
- ASRM classification of müllerian anomalies
- Techniques for pelvic ultrasonography
- Indications for ultrasonography (AIUM)
- Guidelines for examination of pelvic organs
- Ultrasonography of normal uterus
- Uterine abnormalities
- Endometrial abnormalities
- Ultrasonography: Non-neoplastic ovarian lesions
- Ultrasonography features of neoplastic lesions of ovary
- Ultrasonography in acute pelvic pain
- Ultrasonography in chronic pelvic pain
- Conditions where Doppler is useful
- Saline infusion sonography
- Ultrasound-guided procedures
- Ovarian mass
- Algorithm for imaging in abnormal uterine bleeding
- Classification of abnormal uterine bleeding
- Common symptoms in gynecology
- Causes of postmenopausal bleeding
- Clinical evaluation of abnormal uterine bleeding
- Differential diagnosis and investigations of abnormal uterine bleeding
- Causes of vaginal discharge

- Causes of vaginal discharge in reproductive years
- Diagnosis of vaginal infections in reproductive age
- Investigations of vaginal discharge in women during their reproductive years
- Causes of discharge in postmenopausal women
- Clinical evaluation of vaginal discharge in postmenopausal women
- Investigations in postmenopausal women with vaginal discharge
- Evaluation of lower abdominal mass in adolescents
- Lower abdominal masses in reproductive years
- Evaluation of lower abdominal mass during reproductive years
- Evaluation of lower abdominal mass in postmenopausal women
- Evaluation of mass descending per vaginum
- Evaluation of acute lower abdominal/pelvic pain
- Non gynecological causes of acute lower abdominal/pelvic pain
- Acute abdominal pain of gynecological origin
- Evaluation of chronic pelvic pain
- Evaluation of dysmenorrhea
- Common conditions causing pruritus vulvae
- Clinical evaluation of pruritus vulvae
- Causes of dyspareunia and vaginismus
- Clinical evaluation of dyspareunia
- Structural abnormalities of the genital tract causing AUB
- Management of abnormal uterine bleeding in reproductive age group
- History and clinical evaluation of endometrial hyperplasia
- Anatomical classification of myomas
- Subclassification of uterine myoma
- Dimensions of normal ovary
- Benign conditions causing ovarian enlargement
- Ultrasonographic features of benign ovarian lesions

- Management of benign ovarian neoplastic lesions in postmenopausal women
- Management of benign ovarian neoplastic lesions in premenopausal women
- CDC guidelines for diagnosis of acute PID (2015)
- Differential diagnosis of acute PID
- Symptoms and signs of chronic PID.
- Investigations in endometriosis
- Causes of primary amenorrhea
- Evaluation of primary amenorrhea with normal secondary sexual characteristics
- Evaluation of primary amenorrhea with absent secondary sexual characteristics
- Evaluation of secondary amenorrhea

# ABNORMALITIES DUE TO PRESENCE OR ABSENCE OF ANDROGENS AND ANTIMÜLLERIAN HORMONE

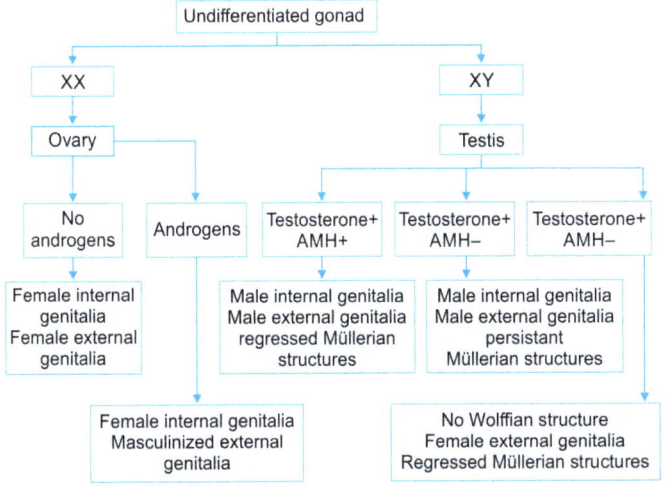

# ASRM CLASSIFICATION OF MÜLLERIAN ANOMALIES

*Class I*

Sequential/complete müllerian agenesis/Aplasia

- Vaginal
- Cervical
- Fundal
- Tubal
- Combined

*Class II*

Unicornuate uterus with/without rudimentary horn

- With rudimentary horn
  - With communicating endometrial cavity
  - Non-communicating cavity
  - With no cavity
- Without rudimentary horn

*Class III*

- Uterine didelphys

*Class IV*

- Bicornuate
  - Complete
  - Partial

*Class V*

- Septate
  - Complete
  - Partial

*Class VI*

- Acute uterus

*Class VII*

- DES related abnormality
  - T-shaped uterus with/without dilated horns

# Common Gynecological Diseases

## TECHNIQUES FOR PELVIC ULTRASONOGRAPHY

- Transabdominal (Curvilinear, 2-5 MHz probe)
  - Full bladder required
  - Panoramic view
  - Useful for large masses
  - Ascites
  - Intra-abdominal organs
  - Lymph nodes
- Transvaginal (Curvilinear 7-12 MHz probe)
  - Bladder should be empty
  - Most useful in gynecology
  - Normal size uterus
    ⇒ Endometrial thickness
    ⇒ Polyps
    ⇒ Growth
  - Normal ovaries, follicles
  - Small masses
  - Pouch of Douglas
- Transperineal
  - Pelvic floor muscles
- Transrectal
  - Puborectalis muscle
  - Anal sphincter
  - Rectovaginal septum

## INDICATIONS FOR ULTRASONOGRAPHY (AIUM)

- Pelvic pain
- Postmenopausal bleeding

- Abnormal uterine bleeding
- Dysmenorrhea
- Abnormal/technically difficult pelvic examination
- Amenorrhea
- Pelvic infection
- Abnormality noted by other imaging
- Infertility
- Congenital anomalies of the genital tract
- Delayed/precocious puberty
- Postoperative pain/bleeding/infection
- Localization of intrauterine contraceptive device (IUCD)
- Screening for cancer in high risk women
- Urinary incontinence/POP
- Preoperative—guidance

## GUIDELINES FOR EXAMINATION OF PELVIC ORGANS

- Uterus
    - Size, shape, orientation
    - Endometrium
    - Myometrium
    - Cervix
- Adnexa
    - Ovaries—size in three dimensions
    - Dilated tubes
    - Mass-size
    - Sonographic characteristics
- Cul-de-sac
    - Fluid
    - Mass—size, position, shape
    - Sonographic characteristics

# ULTRASONOGRAPHY OF NORMAL UTERUS

*Size:* 7.5 × 5.0 × 2.5 cm
*Length:* Fundus to cervix
*Depth:* Anteroposterior

*Myometrium:*
- Homogeneous
- Hypoechogenic

*Endometrium:*
- Changes during menstrual cycle
- 1-4 mm after menstruation
- 8-10 mm at ovulation
- Trilaminar at ovulation

# UTERINE ABNORMALITIES

*Myomas:*
- Irregular uterine contour
- Hypoechoic/isoechoic/hyperechoic masses
- Size, number, location

*Adenomyosis:*
- Uterine enlargement
- Asymmetric thickening
- Heterogeneous echotexture

*Uterine anomalies:*
- Bicornuate/septate uterus
- Hematometra

# ENDOMETRIAL ABNORMALITIES

- Abnormal uterine bleeding
  - Polyps

⇒ Focal lesions
⇒ Hypoechoic/hyperechoic
⇒ Surrounded by endometrial lining
- Submucous leiomyoma
- Postmenopausal bleeding
  - Endometrial thickness
  - Endometrial cancer (myometrial invasion)
- Tamoxifen therapy
  - Increase in thickness
  - Subendometrial stromal vacuolation
- Missing IUCD
  - Bright echogenic
  - Penetration into myometrium
  - Translocation into the peritoneal cavity
- Infertility
  - Endometrial thickness
  - Uterine anomalies

## ULTRASONOGRAPHY: NON-NEOPLASTIC OVARIAN LESIONS

- Infertility
  - Follicular monitoring
  - Dominant follicle 18–20 mm
- Functional cysts
  - Follicular cyst
    ⇒ 3–8 cm, uniloculated
  - Corpus luteum cyst
    ⇒ 3–10 cm, uniloculated
  - Theca lutein cyst
    ⇒ Large, bilateral, multiloculated

- Endometrial cyst
  - Fine low to middle level echoes
  - Ground glass appearance
  - Hyperechoic foci in the wall
  - Rectovaginal modules

## ULTRASONOGRAPHIC FEATURES OF NEOPLASTIC LESIONS OF OVARY

- Serous cystadenoma
  - Cystic
  - Few thin internal septations
- Mucinous cystadenoma
  - Large
  - Multiloculated
  - Each locule with different echogenicity
- Brenner tumor
  - Small
  - Solid
  - Smooth
- Benign cystic teratoma
  - Complex, solid and cystic lesion, calcification, fat fluid levels
  - Echogenic internal components
- Malignant tumors
  - Bilateral
  - Solid/mixed solid and cystic
  - Septae > 3 mm thick
  - Papillary excrescences
  - Thick cyst wall > 3 mm
  - Ascites, omental thickening

- Enlarged para-acoustic nodes
- Liver metastasis

## ULTRASONOGRAPHY IN ACUTE PELVIC PAIN

- Ectopic pregnancy
    - Absence of gestational sac in the uterus
    - Complex adnexal mass
    - Gestational sac in the tube
    - Fetal pole with/without cardiac activity
    - Blood in peritoneal cavity/cul-de-sac (fluid with internal echoes)
- Torsion of ovarian cyst
    - Adnexal mass
    - Cyst with hemorrhage
- Acute PID
    - Inflamed tubes
    - Free fluid in cul-de-sac (anechoic)
    - Pyosalpinx
        ⇒ Pear/retort-shaped tube with anechoic/echogenic fluid
        ⇒ Incomplete septae, fluid debris
        ⇒ Cogwheel appearance
    - Pus in cul-de-sac (echogenic)
    - Tubo-ovarian abscess
        ⇒ Echogenic fluid filled complex mass

## ULTRASONOGRAPHY IN CHRONIC PELVIC PAIN

- Tubo-ovarian mass
    - Complex mass

- Ovary and tube adherent, but can be identified
- Loculated fluid collection around ovary
- Hydrosalpinx
  - Tubular shape
  - Incomplete septae

## CONDITIONS WHERE DOPPLER IS USEFUL

- Torsion of ovarian cyst
- Ectopic pregnancy
- Ovarian malignancy
- Endometrial cancer
- Myoma
- Adenomyosis

## SALINE INFUSION SONOGRAPHY

- Performed preferably on day 5 or 6 of the cycle as an OPD procedure
- To visualize the uterine cavity and diagnose
  - Polyps
  - Submucous myoma
- To test for tubal patency
- Catheter/cannula inserted into the uterus and 5–30 mL sterile saline injected
- Back flow can be prevented by putting a small-sized balloon catheter (8F) and inflating the balloon
- Contraindications
  - Acute PID
  - Hematometra
  - Cervical stenosis

## ULTRASOUND-GUIDED PROCEDURES

- Aspiration of ascitic fluid
- Aspiration of pus/blood for diagnosis of pyoperitoneum/hemoperitoneum
- Drainage of pus/blood from cul-de-sac
- Drainage of pus from abdomen
- Fine-needle aspiration cytology (FNAC) of pelvic/abdominal masses
- Fine-needle aspiration cytology (FNAC) of lymph nodes for diagnosis of tuberculosis and malignancy
- Guided biopsy from abdominal/pelvic masses

## OVARIAN MASS

Algorithm for imaging in ovarian mass.

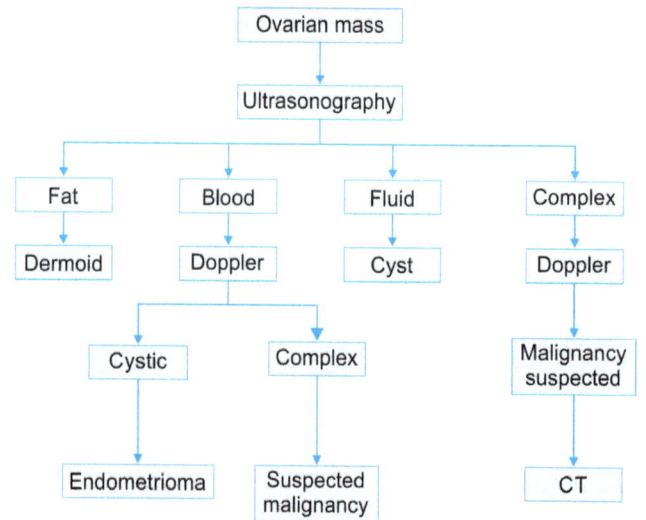

# ALGORITHM FOR IMAGING IN ABNORMAL UTERINE BLEEDING

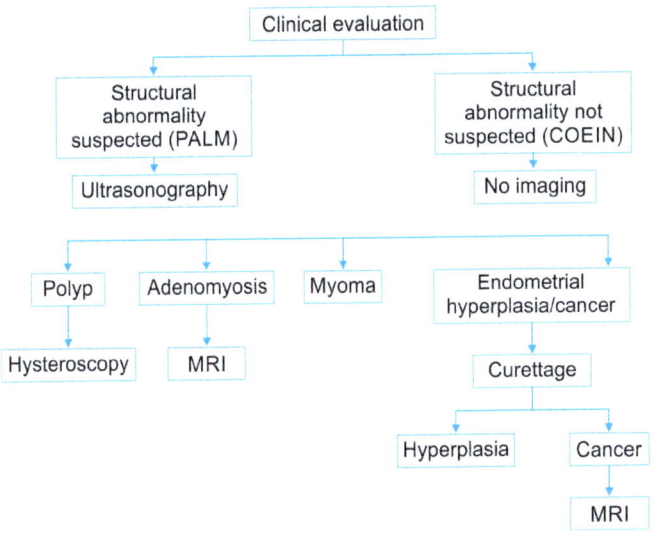

# CLASSIFICATION OF ABNORMAL UTERINE BLEEDING

| PALM | COEIN |
|---|---|
| P—Polyp | C—Coagulopathy |
| A—Adenomyosis | O—Ovulatory dysfunction |
| L—Leiomyoma | E—Endometrial |
| M—Malignancy/hyperplasia | I—Iatrogenic |
|  | N—Not yet classified |

# COMMON SYMPTOMS IN GYNECOLOGY

- Abnormal uterine bleeding
- Vaginal discharge

- Lower abdominal mass
- Mass descending per vaginum
- Acute/chronic pelvic pain
- Dysmenorrhea
- Genital ulcer/swelling/pruritus
- Dyspareunia
- Urinary symptoms
- Bowel symptoms

## CAUSES OF POSTMENOPAUSAL BLEEDING

- Estrogen deficiency vaginitis
- Atrophic endometrium
- Endometrial hyperplasia
- Endometrial polyps
- Endometrial cancer
- Cervical cancer
- Granulosa cell tumor of ovary

## CLINICAL EVALUATION OF ABNORMAL UTERINE BLEEDING

History
- Type of bleeding
- Associated symptoms
    - Preceded by amenorrhea
    - Pelvic pain
    - Dysmenorrhea—congestive/spasmodic
    - Dyspareunia
    - Vaginal discharge

Physical examination
- Abdominal mass
- Speculum examination—polyp, growth
- Bimanual examination
    - Uterine enlargement—regular/irregular
    - Adnexal mass—cystic/solid/mixed, tenderness

## DIFFERENTIAL DIAGNOSIS AND INVESTIGATION OF ABNORMAL UTERINE BLEEDING

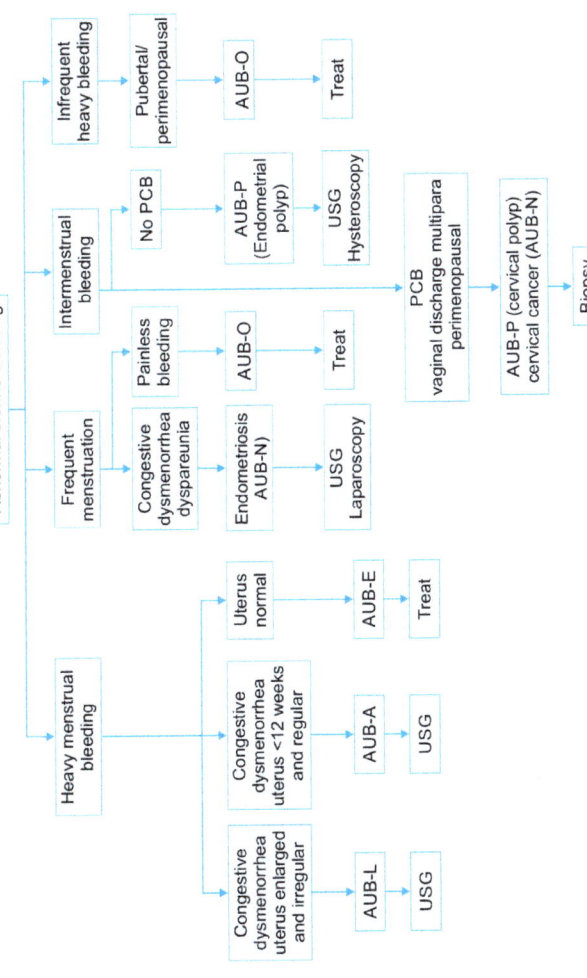

# CAUSES OF VAGINAL DISCHARGE

- Physiological
  - Ovulation
  - Premenstrual
  - During pregnancy
  - Discharge is mucoid, has no odour and is nonirritant
- Pathological
  - Lesions of vagina
  - Lesions of cervix
  - Pelvic inflammatory disease (PID)

**Causes of vaginal discharge in children**

- Nonspecific vulvovaginitis
  - Poor hygiene
  - Allergy
  - Foreign body
- Specific vulvovaginitis
  - *Streptococcus*
  - Other bacteria
  - Pinworm
  - *Candida*
  - *Trichomonas*

# CAUSES OF VAGINAL DISCHARGE IN REPRODUCTIVE YEARS

- Vaginitis
  - Bacterial vaginosis
  - *Trichomonas vaginalis*
  - *Candida* vaginitis
- Cervicitis
  - Gonococcal infection
  - *Chlamydia trachomatis*

- Acute pelvic infection
  - Gonococcal infection
  - *C. trachomatis* infection
- Other pelvic infection
  - Tuberculosis
  - Other infections

# DIAGNOSIS OF VAGINAL INFECTIONS IN REPRODUCTIVE AGE

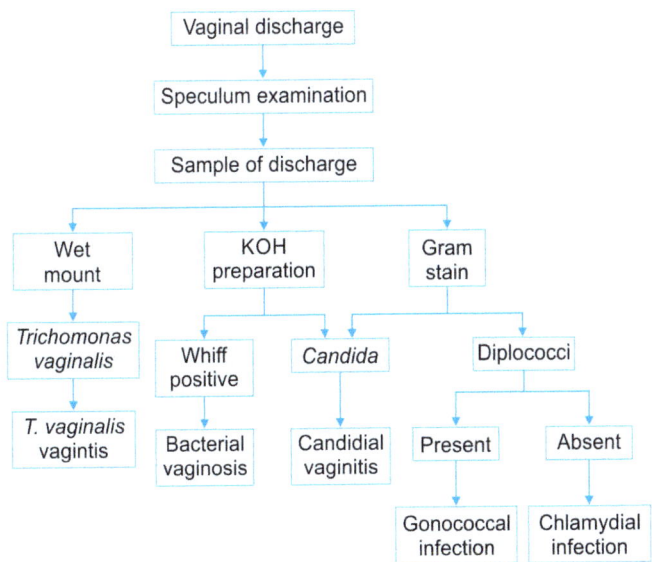

# INVESTIGATIONS OF VAGINAL DISCHARGE IN WOMEN DURING THEIR REPRODUCTIVE YEARS

- Wet film
  - *Trichomonas vaginalis*
  - Clue cells

- KOH preparation
- Whiff test
- Fungal pseudohyphae/spores
- Gram stain
  - Gram-negative diplococci
  - Neutrophils
- Pap smear
- Serology for syphilis
- HIV serology
- Full blood count
  - If PID is suspected

# CAUSES OF DISCHARGE IN POSTMENOPAUSAL WOMEN

| Condition | Clinical features |
|---|---|
| • Estrogen deficiency vaginitis | • Purulent discharge |
|  | • Spotting/bleeding |
| • Cervical cancer | • Foul odour |
|  | • Purulent discharge |
|  | • Blood stained discharge |
|  | • Postcoital staining |
| • Pyometra | • Fever, tachycardia |
|  | • Blood-stained discharge |
|  | • Enlarged, tender, uterus |

# CLINICAL EVALUATION OF VAGINAL DISCHARGE IN POSTMENOPAUSAL WOMEN

i. History
   - Type of discharge

ii. Examination
   - Fever, tachycardia

- Blood-stained or not
- Postmenopausal bleeding
- Postcoital bleeding
- Family history of genital cancer
- Speculum examination
    ⇒ Estrogen deficiency changes
    ⇒ Nature of discharge
    ⇒ Growth on the ectocervix
- Bimanual examination
    ⇒ Endocervical enlargement
    ⇒ Uterine enlargement
    ⇒ Uterine tenderness
    ⇒ Adnexal mass

# INVESTIGATIONS IN POSTMENOPAUSAL WOMEN WITH VAGINAL DISCHARGE

- Pap smear
- Transvaginal ultrasound
    - Endocervical growth
    - Endometrial growth
    - Pyometra
    - Adnexal mass
- Endometrial sampling
- Cervical biopsy

# EVALUATION OF LOWER ABDOMINAL MASS IN ADOLESCENTS

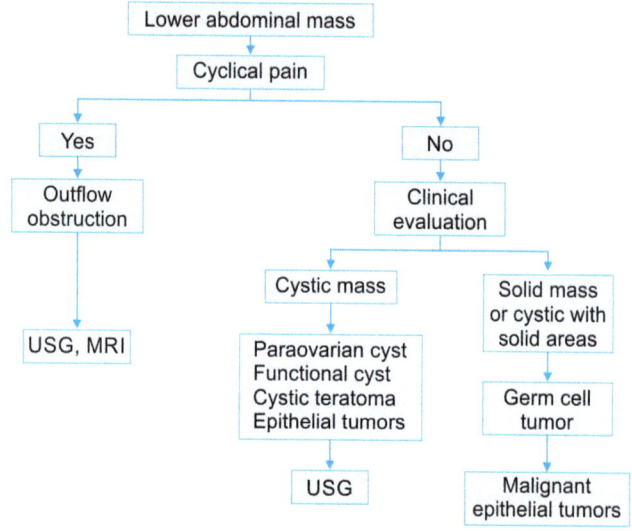

# LOWER ABDOMINAL MASSES IN REPRODUCTIVE YEARS

- Pregnancy
    - Intrauterine
    - Ectopic
    - Vesicular mole
- Uterine
    - Myoma
    - Adenomyoma
- Cervix
    - Myoma
- Mesonephric remnants
    - Paraovarian/paratubal cysts
- Fallopian tube
    - Hydrosalpinx
    - Tubo-ovarian (TO) mass

- Ovary
    - Functional cysts
    - Endometriotic cysts
    - Benign cystic teratoma
    - Serous cystadenoma
    - Mucinous/endometroid/Brenner tumors
    - Malignant
        ⇒ Epithelial tumors
        ⇒ Germ cell tumors

# EVALUATION OF LOWER ABDOMINAL MASS DURING REPRODUCTIVE YEARS

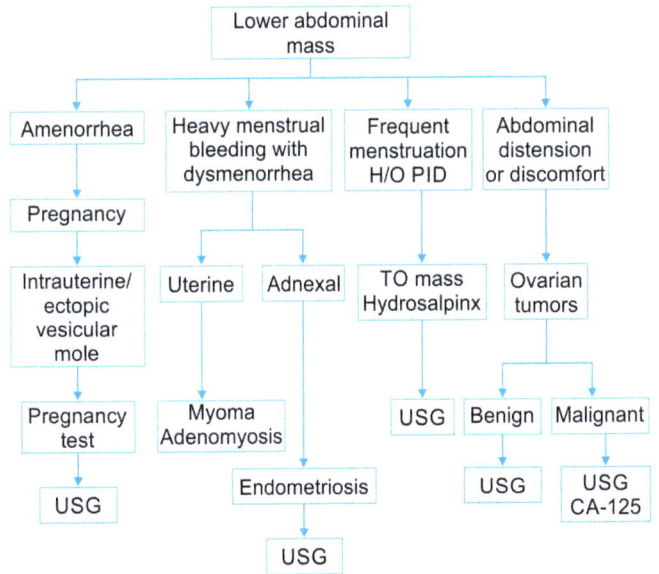

P.S. Other tumors: Lymphoma
Bowel tumor
Bladder tumor

# EVALUATION OF LOWER ABDOMINAL MASS IN POSTMENOPAUSAL WOMEN

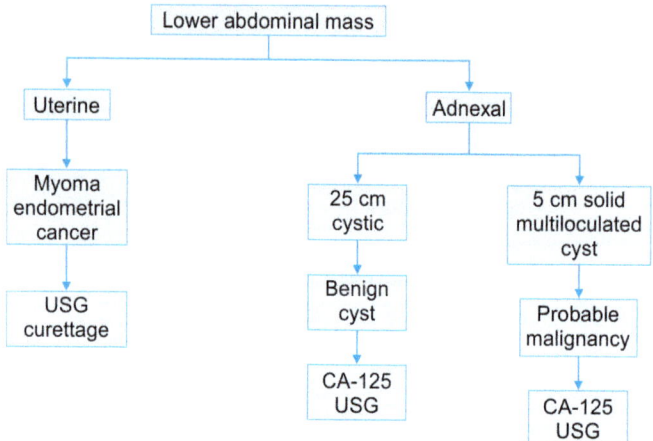

# EVALUATION OF MASS DESCENDING PER VAGINUM

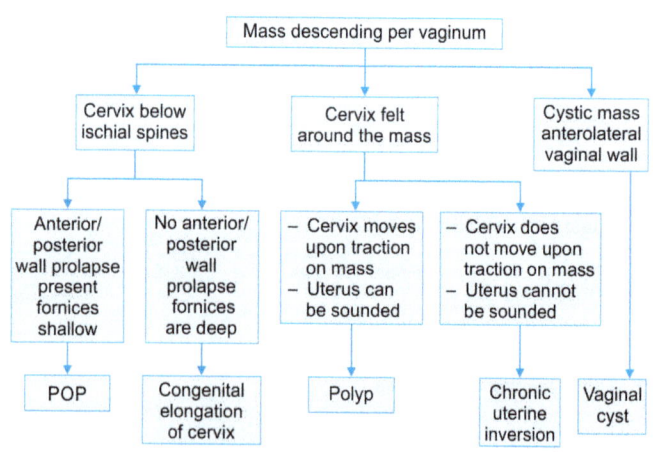

# Common Gynecological Diseases

# EVALUATION OF ACUTE LOWER ABDOMINAL/PELVIC PAIN

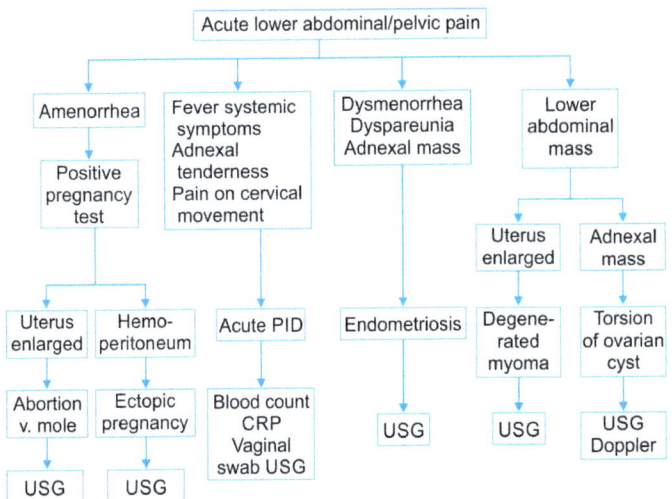

# NONGYNECOLOGICAL CAUSES OF ACUTE LOWER ABDOMINAL/PELVIC PAIN

- Acute appendicitis
- Crohn's disease
- Cystitis
- Ureteric/renal calculus
- Acute cholecystitis
- Perforated peptic ulcer
- Acute pancreatitis
- Mesenteric lymphadenitis

# ACUTE LOWER ABDOMINAL PAIN OF GYNECOLOGICAL ORIGIN

| Condition | Clinical features |
|---|---|
| 1. Abortion | Amenorrhea/uterine enlargement/positive pregnancy test |
| 2. Ectopic pregnancy | Amenorrhea/tender adnexal mass/Hemoperitoneum positive pregnancy test |
| 3. Salpingitis | Fever/systemic signs of sepsis |
| 4. Pyosalpinx/ TO abscess | Adnexal mass/tenderness |
| 5. Red degeneration of myoma | Irregularly enlarged uterus/ history of OCP intake with pregnancy |
| 6. Endometrioma | Dysmenorrhea/dyspareunia/ adnexal mass |
| 7. Torsion of ovarian cyst | Adnexal mass/acute pain/tenderness |
| 8. Rupture of ovarian cyst | Adnexal mass/acute pain |

# Common Gynecological Diseases

## EVALUATION OF CHRONIC PELVIC PAIN

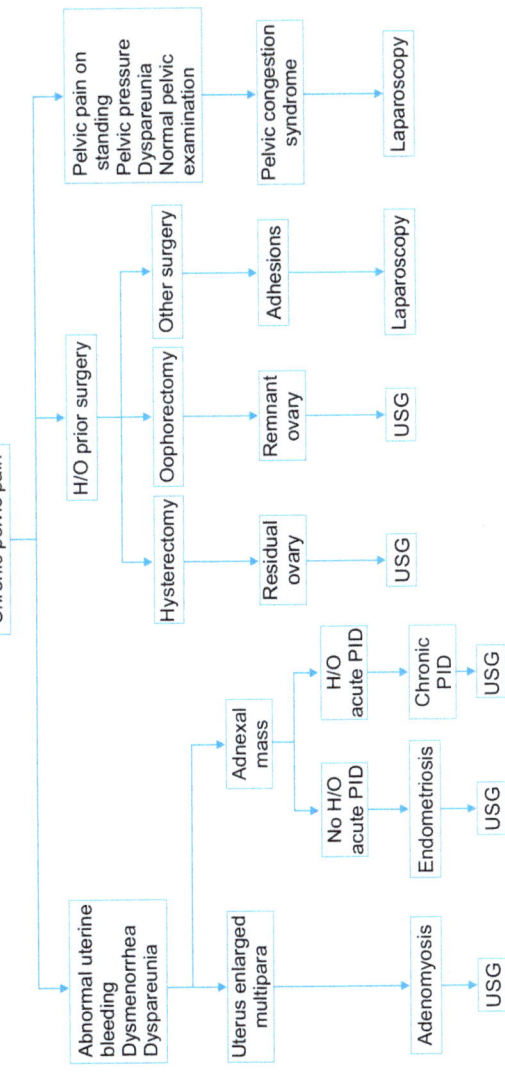

# EVALUATION OF DYSMENORRHEA

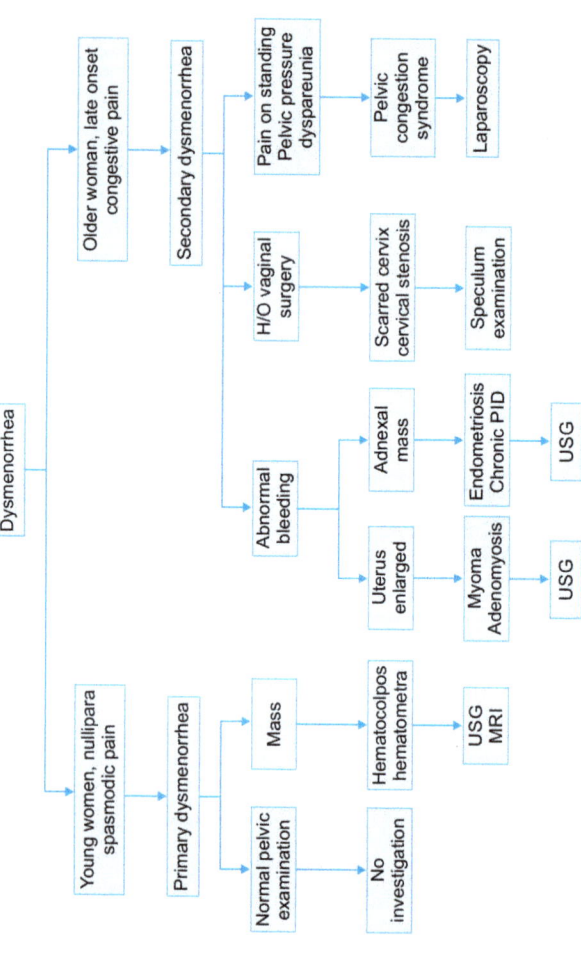

# COMMON CONDITIONS CAUSING PRURITUS VULVAE

- Vulvovaginitis
  - *Candida*
  - Trichomoniasis
  - Gonococcal
  - Bacterial vaginosis
- Dermatitis
  - Seborrhoeic
  - Allergic
  - Primary irritant
  - Atopic
  - Iatrogenic
- Infestation
  - Pediculosis
  - Scabies
- Other conditions
  - Lichen simplex
  - Lichen planus
  - Intertrigo
  - Psoriasis
  - Vulval cancer
  - Paget's disease of the vulva

# CLINICAL EVALUATION OF PRURITUS VULVAE

- History
  - Vaginal discharge
    Color/odour/nature of discharge

- History of allergies
  Atopy/eczema/asthma/contact dermatitis
- Allergens
  Local applications/latex/perfumes
- Family history
  Psoriasis/allergies
- History of systemic illnesses
  Diabetes/Crohn's disease
- Physical examination
  - General examination
    Psoriasis/seborrhea/lichen planus
  - Examination of vulva
    Skin lesions/pigmentation/excoriation/discharge
  - Speculum examination
    Discharge
  - Bimanual examination
    Evidence of pelvic inflammatory disease

# CAUSES OF DYSPAREUNIA AND VAGINISMUS

- Superficial dyspareunia/vaginismus
  - Vaginitis—*Candida/Trichomonas/Gonococcus*
  - Vulvar lesions—Lichen planus/lichen sclerosis/dermatitis
  - Vulvodynia
  - Vulvar vestibulitis
  - Lichen sclerosis
  - Prior episiotomy/surgery
  - Postmenopausal estrogen deficiency

- Postradiation scarring
- Psychogenic—Sexual abuse/lack of sexual interest
- Deep dyspareunia
    - Endometriosis
    - Chronic PID
    - Ovaries prolapsed in the pouch of Douglas
    - Acutely retroverted uterus
    - Adnexal pathology

## CLINICAL EVALUATION IN DYSPAREUNIA

- History
    - Timing of pain in relation to intercourse
    - Vaginal discharge
    - Dyspareunia
    - Menopause
    - Prior surgery/radiation
    - Prior sexual abuse
    - Anxiety/depression
- Physical examination
    - General examination
    Depression/anxiety
    - Local examination
    Vulval lesions/excoriation
    - Speculum examination
    Spasm of muscles/discharge/scarring/dryness/signs of vaginitis
    - Bimanual examination
    Retroverted uterus/mobility/adnexal mass/induration of uterosacrals

# STRUCTURAL ABNORMALITIES OF THE GENITAL TRACT CAUSING AUB

| Abnormality polyp | Age group | Type of bleeding |
|---|---|---|
| • Endometrial polyp | Reproductive age<br><br>Postmenopausal | • Heavy menstrual bleeding<br>• Intermenstrual bleeding<br>• Postmenopausal bleeding |
| • Cervical polyp | Reproductive age | • Intermenstrual bleeding<br>• Postcoital bleeding |
| • Adenomyosis | Perimenopausal | Heavy menstrual bleeding |
| *Leiomyoma* | | |
| • Submucosal | Reproductive age<br><br>Postmenopausal | • Heavy menstrual bleeding<br>• Intermenstrual bleeding<br>• Heavy menstrual bleeding |
| • Intramural | Reproductive | • Heavy menstrual bleeding<br>• Irregular bleeding |
| *Malignancy/hyperplasia* | | |
| • Endometrium<br><br><br>• Cervical | Postmenopausal<br><br>Perimenopausal<br><br>Premenopausal | • Postmenopausal bleeding<br>• Heavy menstrual bleeding<br>• Irregular bleeding<br>• Intermenstrual bleeding<br>• Postcoital bleeding |

# Common Gynecological Diseases

## MANAGEMENT OF ABNORMAL UTERINE BLEEDING IN REPRODUCTIVE AGE GROUP

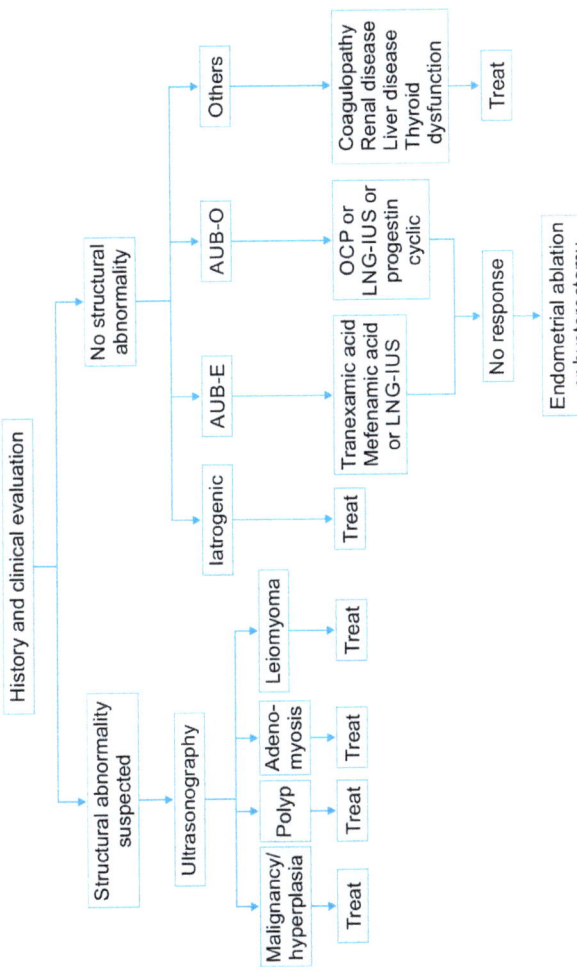

# HISTORY AND CLINICAL EVALUATION OF ENDOMETRIAL HYPERPLASIA

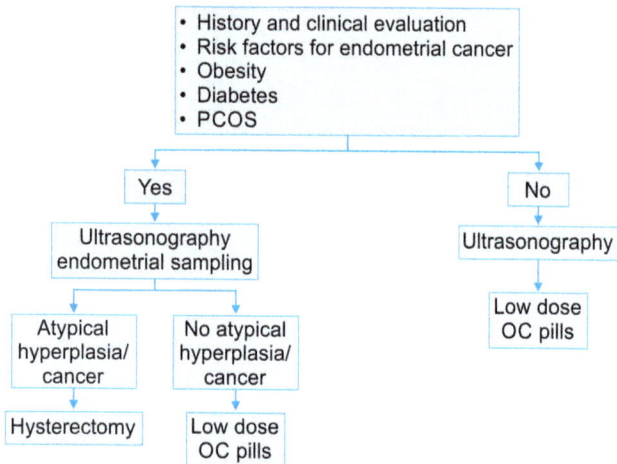

# ANATOMICAL CLASSIFICATION OF MYOMAS

- Myomas in the body of the uterus
  - Subserosal
  - Intramural
  - Submucosal
- Cervical myomas
  - Anterior
  - Posterior
  - Central
- Broad ligament myomas
  - *True:* Arising from smooth muscle in the broad ligament
  - *Pseudo:* Arising from the uterus and projecting into broad ligament

# SUBCLASSIFICATION OF UTERINE MYOMA

SM—Submucosal

    *0:* Pedunculated, lies entirely within the uterine cavity

*1:* <50% intramural
*2:* >50% intramural

O—Other

*3:* Contacts endometrium, 100% intramural
*4:* Intramural
*5:* Subserosal >50% intramural
*6:* Subserosal <50% intramural
*7:* Subserosal pedunculated
*8:* Other (cervical, broad ligament)

## DIMENSIONS OF NORMAL OVARY

- Premenopausal ovary
  *Size:* $3 \times 2 \times 2$ cm$^3$
  *Volume:* 10 cm$^3$
  Upper limit of normal 18 cm$^3$
- Postmenopausal ovary
  *Size:* $2 \times 1.5 \times 1$ cm$^3$
  *Volume:* 3 cm$^3$
  Upper limit of normal 8 cm$^3$

## BENIGN CONDITIONS CAUSING OVARIAN ENLARGEMENT

- Functional cysts
  - Follicular cysts
  - Corpus luteum cysts
  - Theca lutein cysts
- Benign neoplasms
  - Epithelial cells tumors
  - Germ cell tumors
  - Stromal tumors
- Others
  - Endometrioma
  - Ovarian hyperstimulation syndrome (PCOS)
  - Ovarian hyperstimulation syndrome (OHSS)

## ULTRASONOGRAPHIC FEATURES OF BENIGN OVARIAN LESIONS

- *Size:* <8 cm, ovarian volume: <10 cm$^3$
- Cystic lesions
- No solid areas
- No papillary excrescences
- Thin walled (<3 mm)
- Uniloculated
- If multiloculated, thin septal (<2 mm)
- Unilateral
- No ascites/retroperitoneal nodules
- No metastasis

## MANAGEMENT OF BENIGN OVARIAN NEOPLASTIC LESIONS IN POSTMENOPAUSAL WOMEN

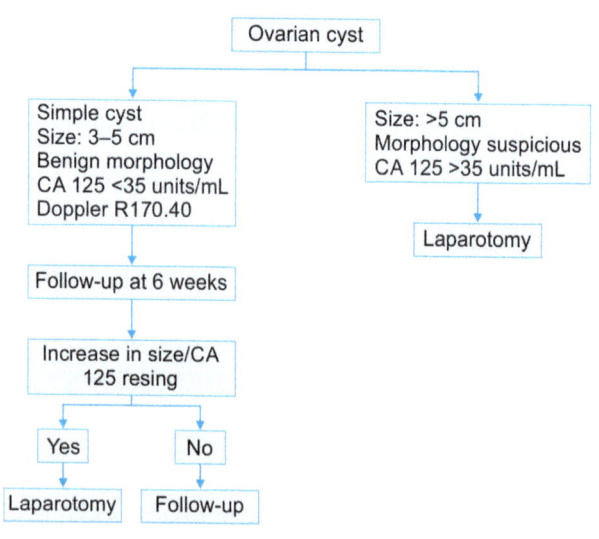

# Common Gynecological Diseases

## MANAGEMENT OF BENIGN OVARIAN NEOPLASTIC LESIONS IN PREMENOPAUSAL WOMEN

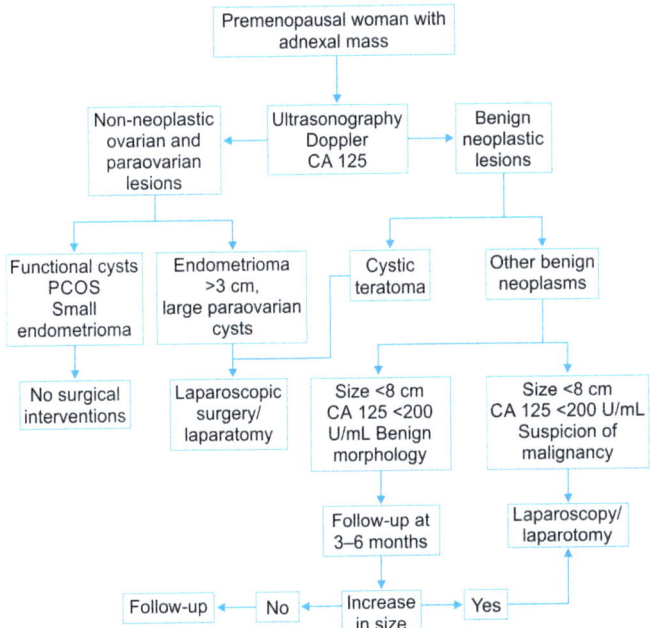

## CDC GUIDELINES FOR DIAGNOSIS OF ACUTE PID (2015)

- Minimum criteria
  - Uterine tenderness
  - Adnexal tenderness
  - Cervical motion tenderness
- Additional criteria for diagnosis
  - Oral temperature > 38°C

- Abnormal cervical mucopurulent discharge or cervical friability
- *Vaginal discharge:* WBC's on microscopy
- Laboratory documentation of cervical infection with *N. gonorrhoeae* or *Chlamydia trachomatis*
- Elevated ESR
- Elevated C-reactive protein
- Definitive criteria for diagnosis of PID
  - Endometrial biopsy
    ⇒ Histopathological evidence of endometritis
  - Transvaginal ultrasonogram/MRI
    ⇒ Thickened tube
    ⇒ Fluid filled tubes
    ⇒ Tubo-ovarian mass
  - Doppler studies suggestive of pelvic infection
  - Laparoscopy
    ⇒ Tubal erythema, edema, adhesions
    ⇒ Pyosalpinx/tubo-ovarian mass
    ⇒ Purulent exudates in POD

## DIFFERENTIAL DIAGNOSIS OF ACUTE PID

- Gynecological conditions
  - Ectopic pregnancy
  - Torsion/rupture of ovarian cyst
  - Endometriosis
- Nongynecological conditions
  - Acute appendicitis
  - Diverticulitis
  - Irritable bowel syndrome
  - Inflammatory bowel syndrome
  - Urinary tract infection
  - Functional pain

# SYMPTOMS AND SIGNS OF CHRONIC PID

| Symptoms | Signs |
|---|---|
| • History of previous infection<br>• Lower abdominal pain<br>• Deep dyspareunia<br>• Congestive dysmenorrhea<br>• Menstrual abnormalities<br>  ▪ Heavy menstrual bleeding<br>  ▪ Frequent menstruation<br>• Low backache<br>• Chronic pelvic pain<br>• Infertility | • Abdominal examination<br>  ▪ Tenderness<br>  ▪ Mass arising from the pelvis<br>• Per speculum examination<br>  ▪ Vaginal/cervical discharge may be present<br>• Pelvic examination<br>• Fixed, retroverted, tender uterus<br>• Adnexal tenderness<br>• Pelvic mass<br>  ▪ Hydrosalpinx<br>  ▪ Tubo-ovarian mass<br>• Frozen pelvis |

# INVESTIGATION IN ENDOMETRIOSIS

- Ultrasound—Abdominal/transvaginal
  - Not useful in superficial endometriosis
  - Not accurate in deep infiltrating endometriosis
  - Useful in ovarian endometrioma
    ⇒ Ovarian mass
      – Cystic mass
      – Low level internal echoes
      – Hyperechoic foci in the wall
    ⇒ Hydroureteronephrosis
- Magnetic resonance imaging
  - Not useful in superficial endometriosis
  - Less accurate in deep infiltrating endometriosis
  - Useful in ovarian endometriosis

- ⇒ Endometrioma larger than 1 cm
- ⇒ Rectovaginal nodules
- Doppler ultrasound
  Not very useful
- Barium studies
  In severe bowel endometriosis
- Intravenous urography
  - Severe endometriosis
  - Suspected ureteric involvement

## CAUSES OF PRIMARY AMENORRHEA

- Hypothalamic-pituitary functioning
  a. Congenital
    - Isolated GnRH deficiency
    - Multiple pituitary hormone deficiencies
  b. Acquired
    - Hydrocephalus
      ⇒ Infections
      ⇒ Trauma
      ⇒ Empty sella syndrome
      ⇒ Tumors
    - Functional hypothalamic amenorrhea
      ⇒ Anorexia nervosa
      ⇒ Exercise
      ⇒ Stress
- Ovarian dysgenesis
  - Turner syndrome and its variants
  - XX/XY gonadal agenesis
- Uterus
  - Uterovaginal agenesis
  - Menstrual outflow obstruction

# Common Gynecological Diseases

- Adrenal
  - Congenital adrenal hyperplasia
    ⇒ 17α hydroxylase deficiency
  - Androgen secreting tumors
- Thyroid
  - Prepubertal/Juvenile hypothyroidism
- Others
  - Androgen insensitivity syndrome
  - 5α reductase deficiency
  - Constitutional delay
  - Prior chemotherapy or radiotherapy

## EVALUATION OF PRIMARY AMENORRHEA WITH NORMAL SECONDARY SEXUAL CHARACTERISTICS

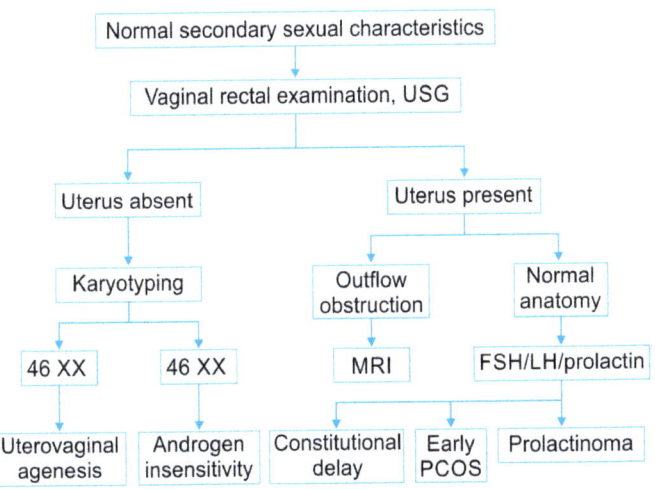

# EVALUATION OF PRIMARY AMENORRHEA WITH ABSENT SECONDARY SEXUAL CHARACTERISTICS

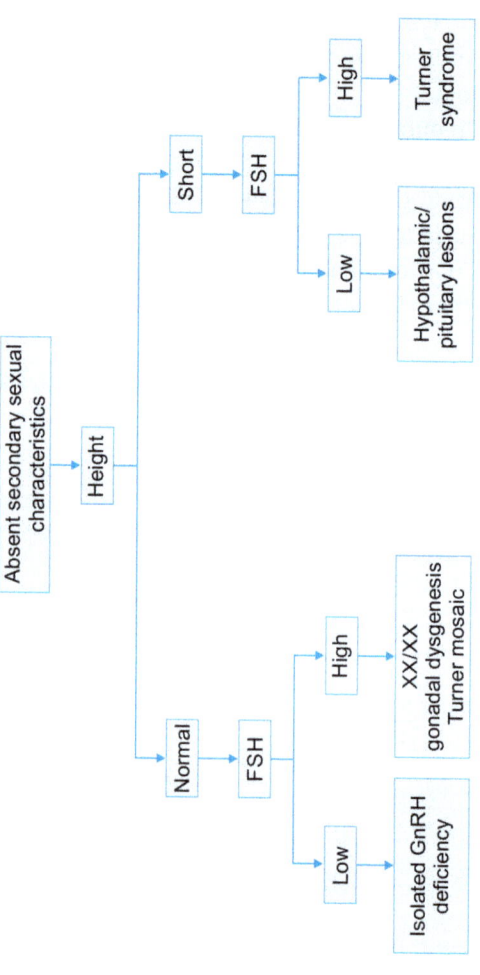

# Common Gynecological Diseases

## EVALUATION OF SECONDARY AMENORRHEA

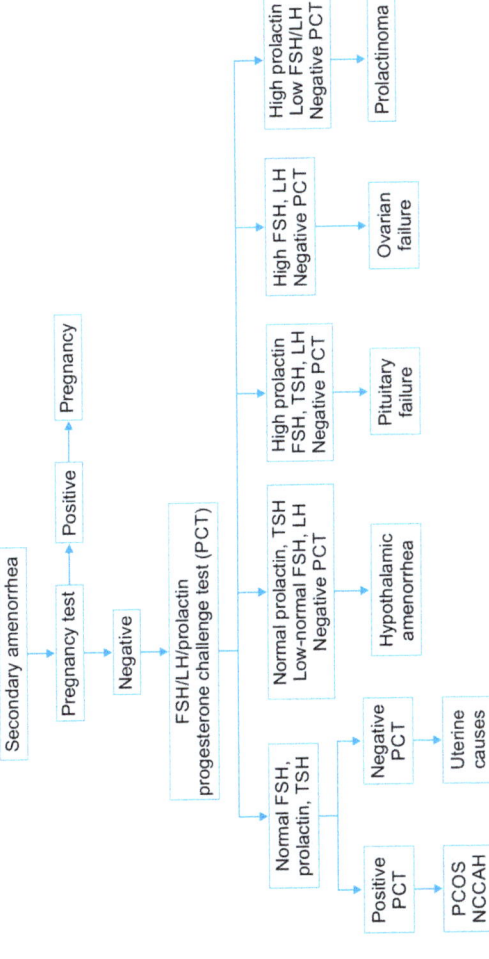

## GENETIC DEVELOPMENT IN FEMALES

**Flowchart 15.1:** Common gynecological diseases and an approach to diagnosis.

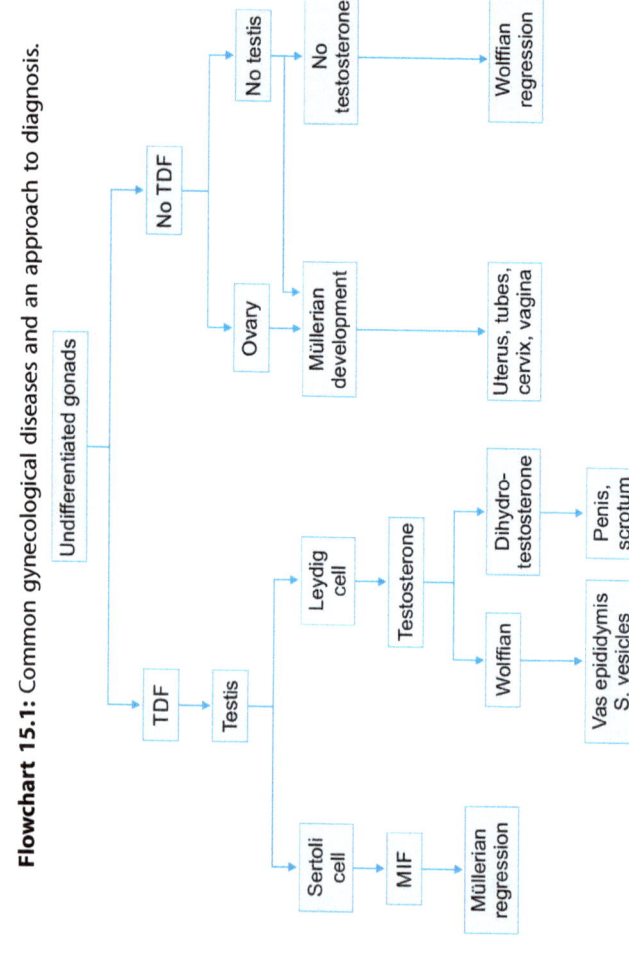

## Common Gynecological Diseases

**Flowchart 15.2:** Genetic abnormalities.

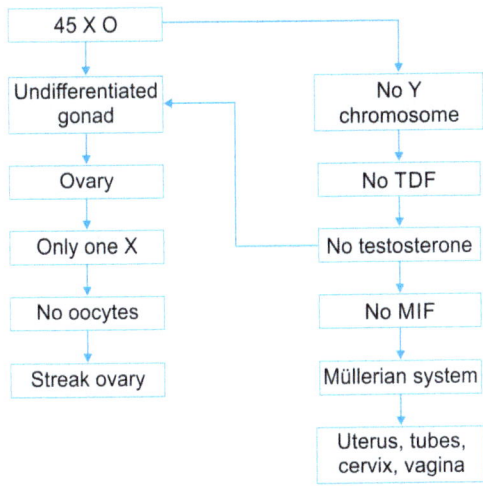

**Flowchart 15.3:** XY gonadal agenesis.

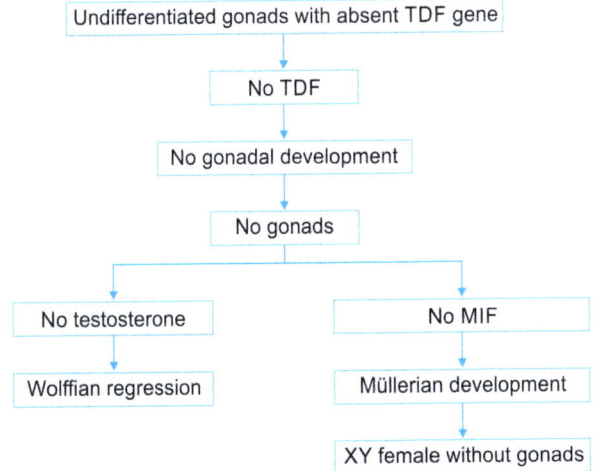

## Ultrasound in Gynecology

**Flowchart 15.4:** USG approach to suspected ectopic.

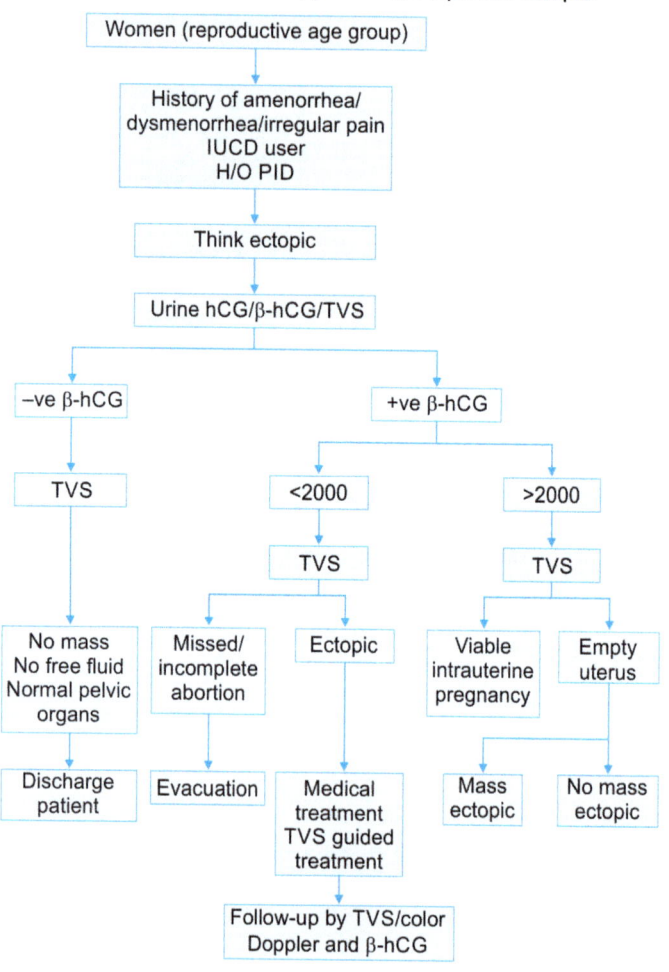

# Common Gynecological Diseases

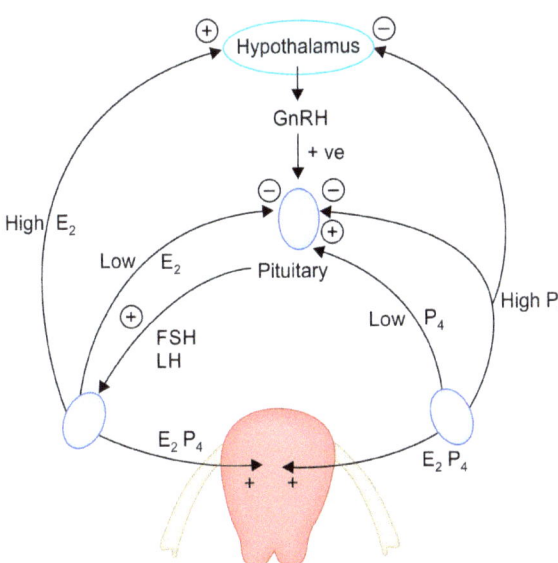

**Fig. 15.1:** Hypothalamopituitary-ovarian axis

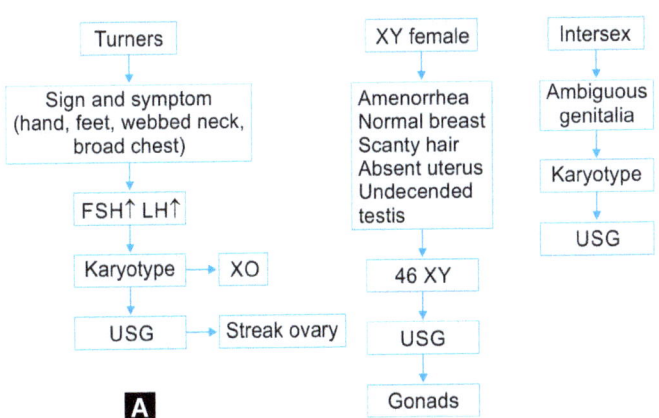

**Fig. 15.2A**

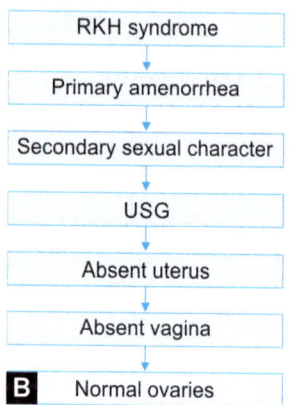

**Figs. 15.2A and B:** (A) Approach to diagnosis. (B) Vaginal atresia.

**Flowchart. 15.5:** USG approach to DUB.

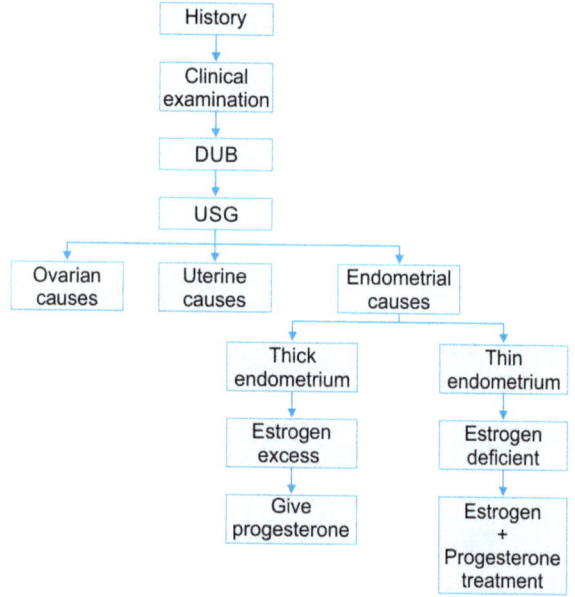

# Common Gynecological Diseases

**Flowchart 15.6:** An ultrasound approach to menstrual problems.

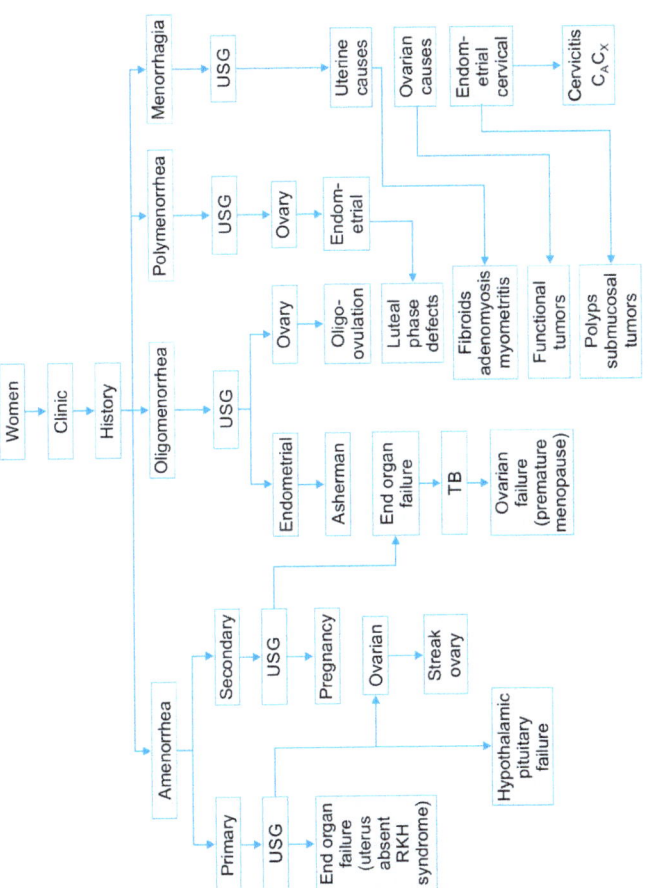

**Flowchart 15.7:** Dilation and curettage.

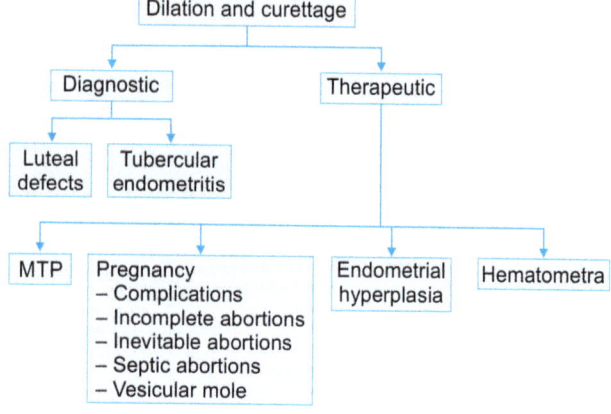

**Flowchart 15.8:** Approach to vaginal bleeding.

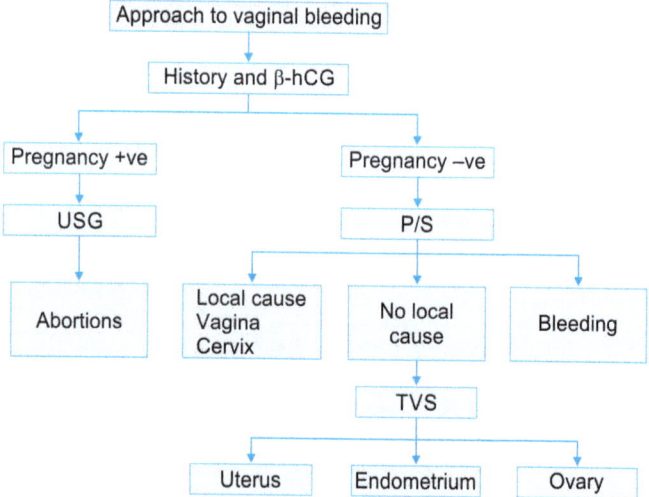

## Common Gynecological Diseases

**Flowchart 15.9:** Approach to gynecological pain.

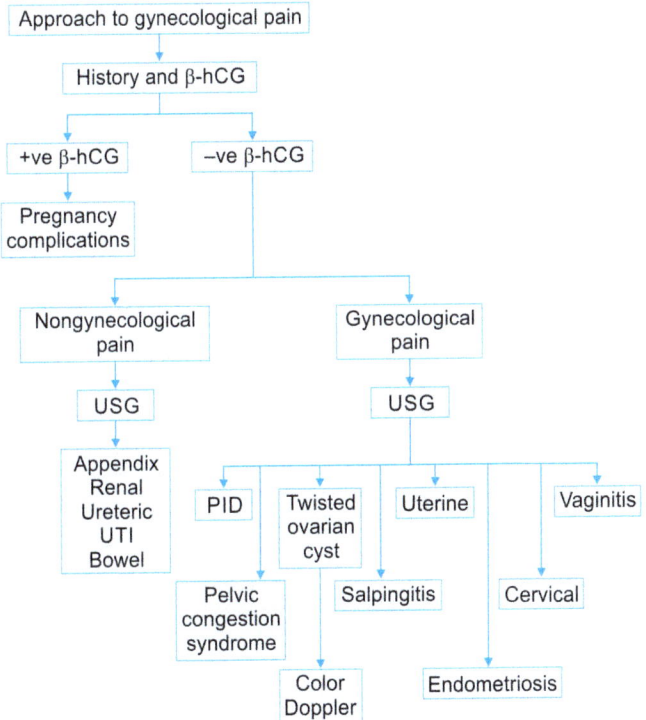

## Flowchart 15.10: Ectopic pregnancy.

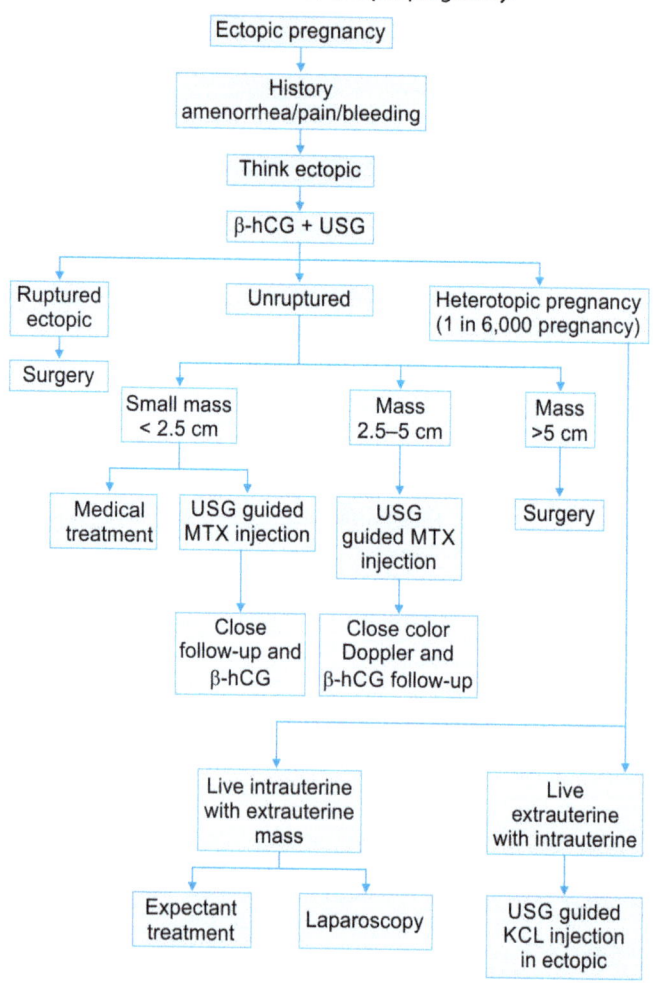

## Common Gynecological Diseases

**Flowchart 15.11:** Polycystic/multicystic ovaries.

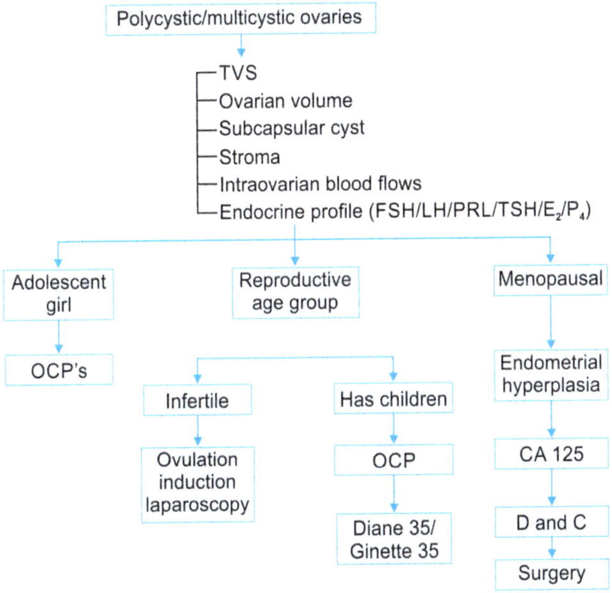

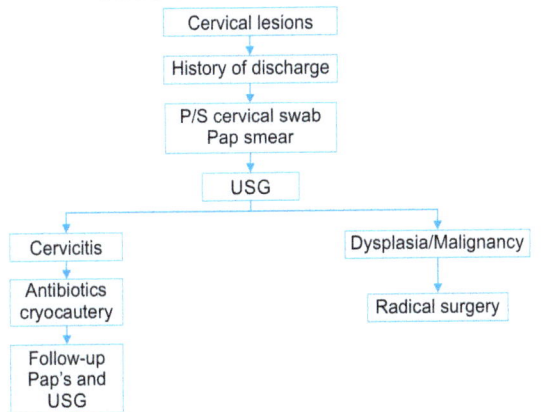

**Flowchart 15.12:** Cervical lesions.

**Flowchart 15.13:** Endometrial hyperplasia.

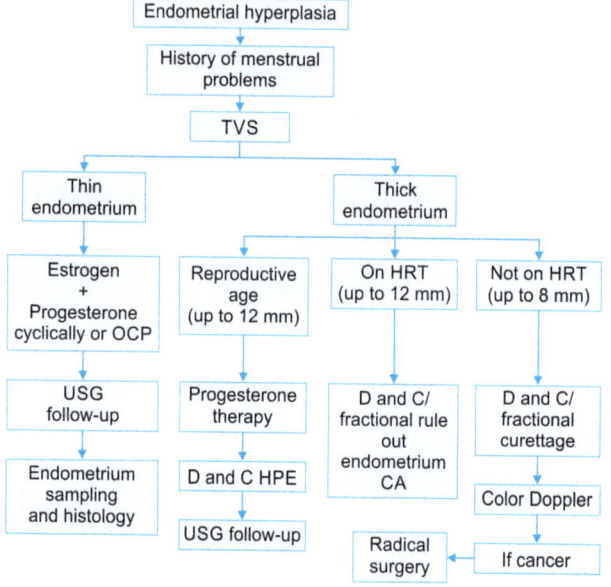

**Flowchart 15.14:** Pelvic inflammatory disease.

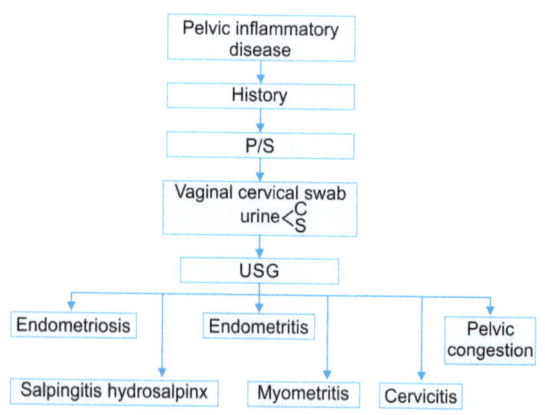

## Common Gynecological Diseases

**Flowchart 15.15:** Simple ovarian follicular cyst.

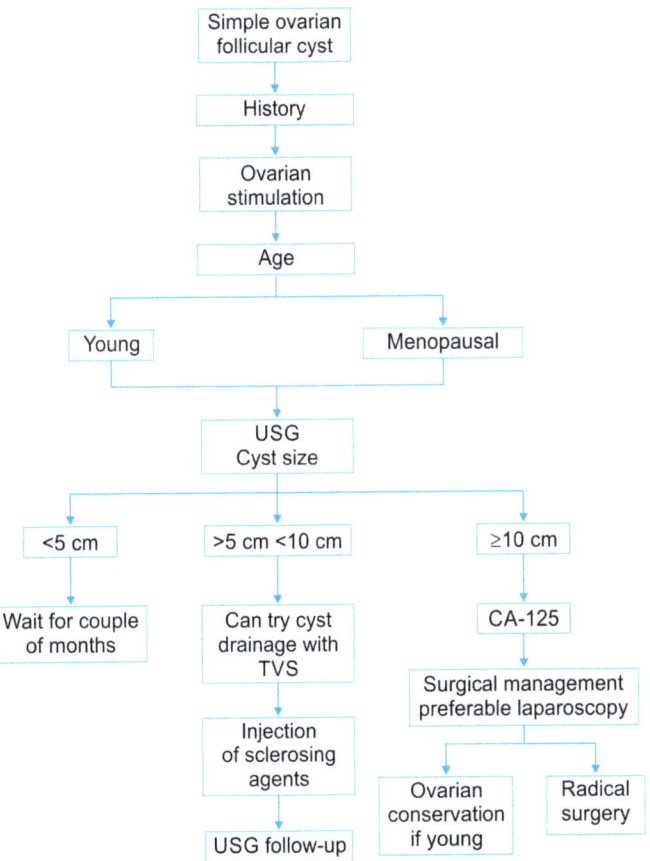

**Flowchart 15.16:** Ultrasound screening for ovarian neoplasms.

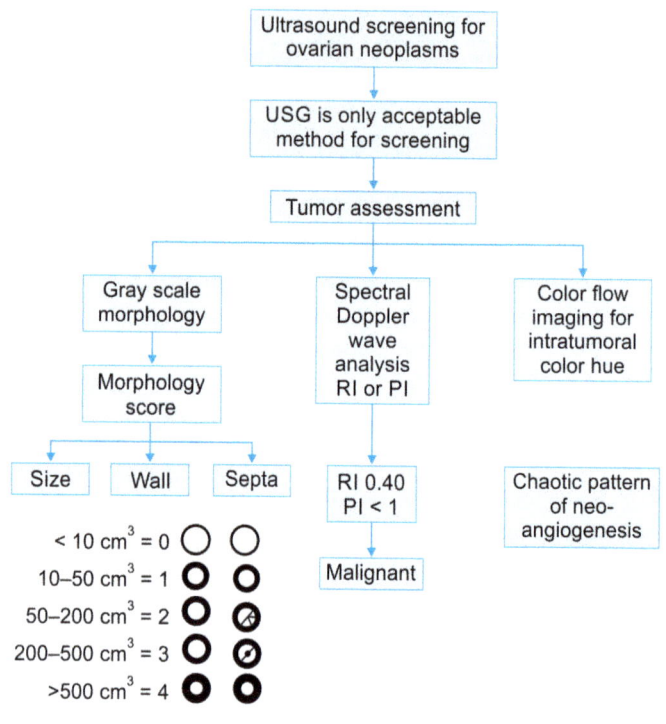

# Common Gynecological Diseases

**Flowchart 15.17:** Sonographic evaluation of fibroids.

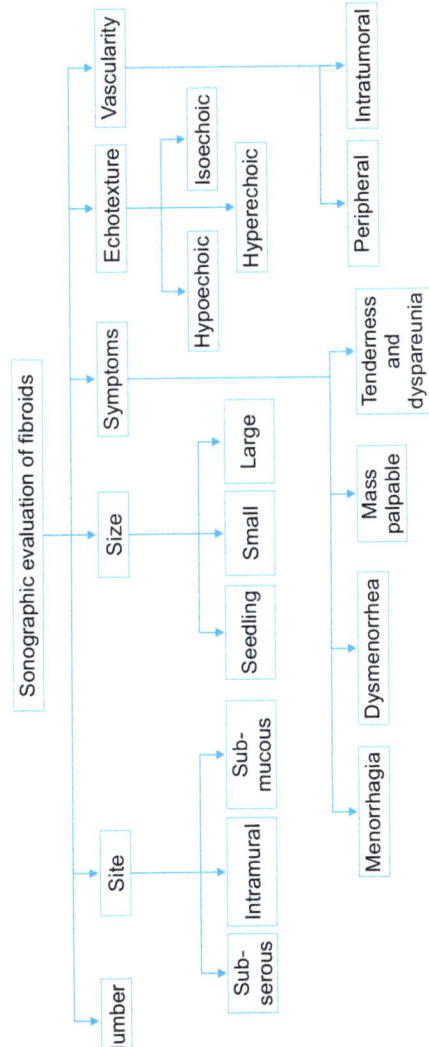

**Flowchart 15.18:** Approach to menopausal problems.

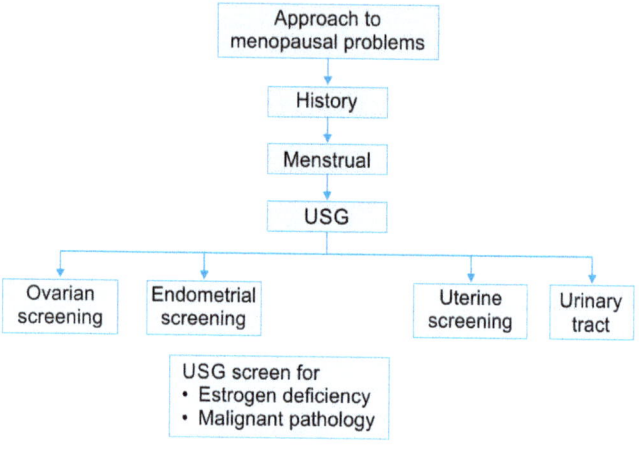

**Flowchart 15.19:** Ovarian tumor.

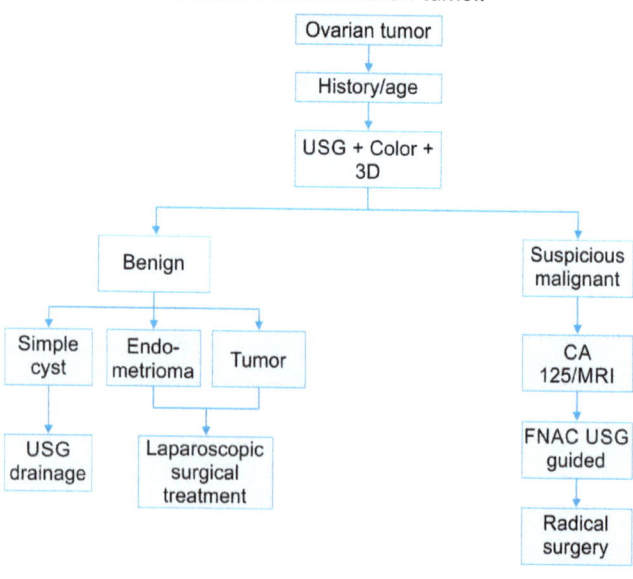

## Common Gynecological Diseases

**Flowchart 15.20:** Endometriosis.

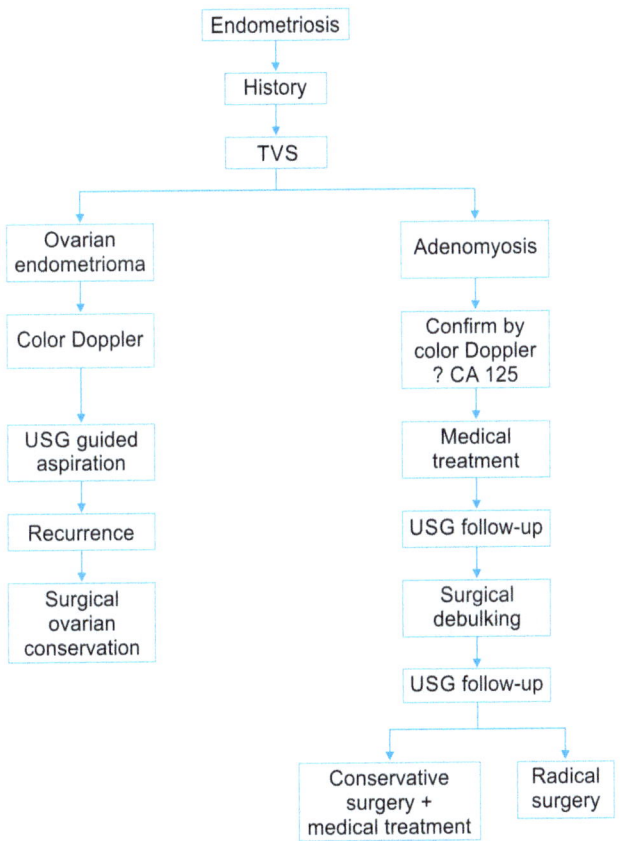

## Ultrasound in Gynecology

**Flowchart 15.21:** Postmenopausal bleeding.

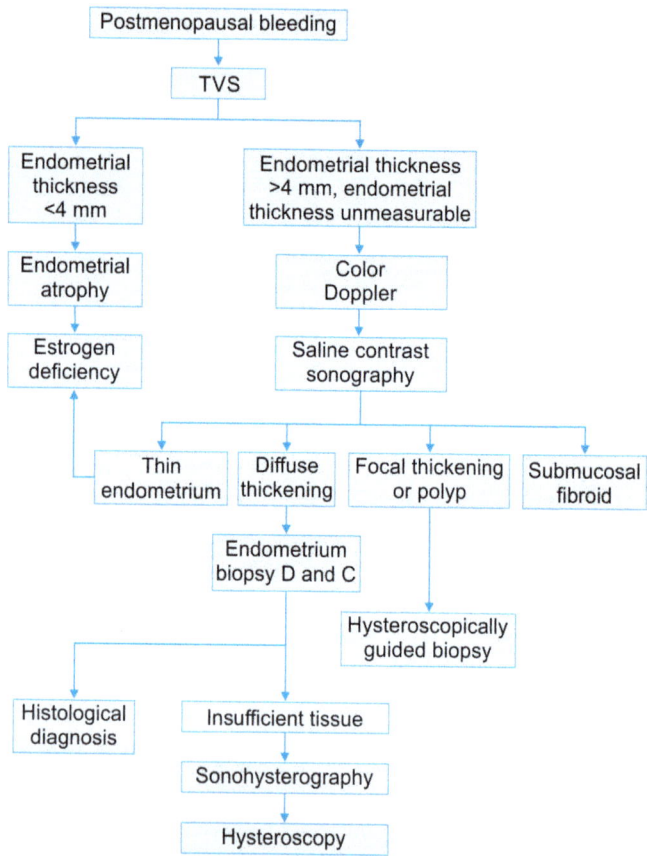

## Common Gynecological Diseases

**Flowchart 15.22:** Ultrasound evaluation of infertility.

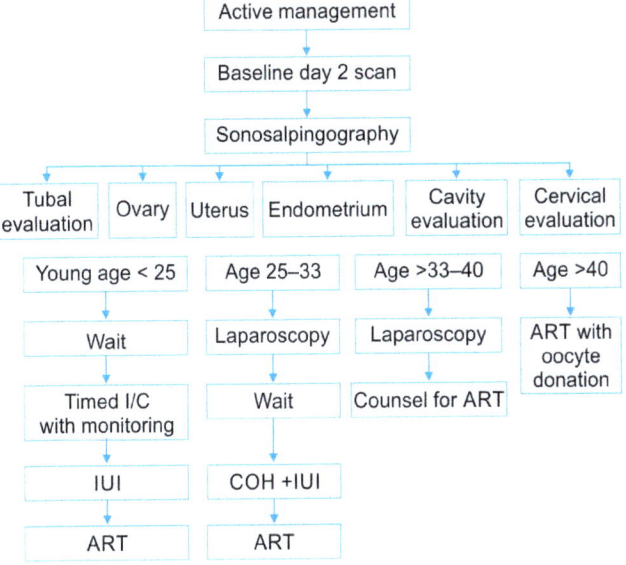

**Flowchart 15.23:** ART protocol.

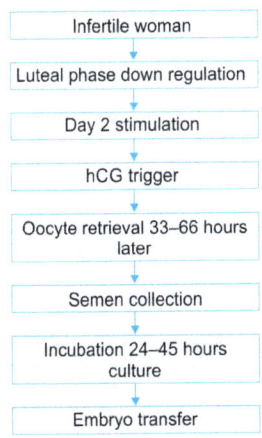

# APPENDIX

## Measurement

### Uterine Size

- *Prepuberty uterus*: 1-3 cm in length, 0.5-1 cm in AP diameter, 0.5-1 cm in width
- *Nulliparous uterus*: 6-8.5 cm in length, 2-4 cm in AP diameter, 3-5 cm in width
- *Multiparous uterus*: 8-10 cm in length, 3-5 cm in AP diameter, 4-6 cm in width
- *Postmenopausal uterus*: 3.5-7.5 cm in length, 1.7-3.3 cm in AP diameter, 2-4 cm in width

### Ovarian Size

- *In children:* 2-3 cc in volume
- *In adolescent:* 4-5 cc in volume
- *In adults:* 6-8 cc in volume
- *At menopause:* 3-7 cc

| Endometrial thickness | Depends on menstrual age |
|---|---|
| $D_1$–$D_5$ (menstrual phase) | <4 mm (2–3 mm) appears as hyperechoic line |
| $D_6$–$D_{10}$ (early proliferative phase) | 4–6 mm, hypoechoic |
| $D_{11}$–$D_{14}$ (preovulatory phase) | 6–10 mm, triple line pattern seen |
| Postovulatory/transitory phase | 8–14 mm, hyperechoic |
| Postmenopause | <4 mm, thin hyperechoic |
| Postmenopausal women in HRT | 4–8 mm thickness, variable USG pattern |

# Index

Page numbers followed by *f* refer to figure, *fc* refer to flowchart, and *t* refer to table.

## A

Abdominal examination 240, 277
Abnormal uterine bleeding 241, 246, 247, 253
   classification of 241, 253
   clinical evaluation of 241, 254
   differential diagnosis of 241, 255
   investigations of 241, 255
   management of 242, 272
Abortion 264
   missed 136
   previous 185
Abruptio placenta 47
Abscess 264
Absorption 5
Acute lower abdominal pain
   evaluation of 242
   non-gynecological causes of 242, 263
Acute pelvic inflammatory disease 187, 192*f*, 250, 251
   diagnosis of 243, 275
   differential diagnosis of 243, 276
   history of 234
Acute pelvic pain 254
   ultrasonography in 241, 250
Adenomyoma 260
Adenomyosis 97, 113, 228, 229, 233, 234, 240, 247, 251, 253, 270
Adhesions 234, 235, 240
Adnexa 58, 246

Adnexal mass 154, 222, 250, 254, 259, 264
Adnexal pathology 269
Adnexal tenderness 240, 277
Adrenal hyperplasia, congenital 279
Allergens 235
Allergy 256
Amenorrhea 195, 197, 246, 254, 264
American Fertility Society Classification 139
Amniotic fluid, reduced 213
Anal sphincter 245
Androgen 241, 243
   insensitivity syndrome 279
   secreting tumors 279
Anemia 212
Anorexia nervosa 278
Anovulation 165
Anteflexion 75
Anterior wall
   submucous fibroid 109*f*
   subserous fibroids 105*f*
Anteversion 75
Antimüllerian hormone 241, 243
Anxiety 233, 269
Appendicitis, acute 263, 276
Arcuate artery calcification, multiple foci of 71*f*
Ascites 245
Ascitic fluid, aspiration of 252
Asherman's syndrome 143*f*, 151

Assisted reproductive
    technique 185
    protocol 299*fc*
Atrophy 229
Audible sound waves 1
Audio volume 34

# B

Bacterial vaginosis 256
Basal layer 76
Battery injury 43
Beam profile 6
Benign ovarian
    lesions, ultrasonographic
        features of 242, 274
    neoplastic lesions, management
        of 243, 274, 275
Beta hCG 196
    level, correlation of 197
Bimanual examination 254, 269
Biopsy, endometrial 276
Bladder tumor 261
Bleeding 246
    types of 270
Blob sign 203
Blood
    flow velocity 23*f*
    pressure, elevated 212
Bowel 190
    symptoms 239, 254
    tumor 261
Breast
    cancer 47
    cyst 47
Brenner tumor 249, 261
Broad ligament myomas 272

# C

Calcifications 97
Cancer, endometrial 224, 248, 251, 254

Candida 268
    vaginitis 256
Carcinoma, endometrial 133
Cavity
    abdominal 197
    endometrial 98*f*, 108*f*, 244
Cervical
    biopsy 259
    canal 99*f*, 180*f*
    cancer 118*f*, 254, 258
    carcinoma 183
    disorders 179
    ectopic pregnancy 198
    fibroid 179
    lesions 291*fc*
    myomas 272
    polyp 182, 270
    pregnancy 183, 204
    stenosis 183, 251
Cervicitis 256
Cervix 59, 117*f*, 205*f*, 260
    lesions of 256
    normal 95*f*, 180*f*
Cesarean section scar 227
Chemotherapy 279
Chlamydia 240
    trachomatis 256
Cholecystitis, acute 263
Chronic pelvic inflammatory
        disease 232, 233, 269
    signs of 243, 277
    symptoms of 243, 277
Chronic pelvic pain 230, 230*t*, 239*t*,
        240*t*, 254, 277
    causes of 233*t*, 236*t*
    evaluation of 231*fc*, 242, 265
    gynecological causes of 234*t*
    management of 231*fc*
    ultrasonography in 241, 250
    urological causes of 235*t*
Clue cells 257
Cogwheel appearance 250
Color Doppler 162

Color flash 38
Color flow 97
    baseline 32
    display 30
    imaging 30
    mapping 178
    pattern 204
Color inversion 32
Color misregistration artifact 38
Comparative power output test 42
Complete blood count 240
Complex adnexal mass 250
Compression elastography 18
Conception, retained products
    of 225
Continuous-wave Doppler 23
Copper-containing devices 216
Cornual pregnancy, ruptured 198
Corpus luteal cyst 203*f*
Corpus luteum 203
    cyst 89*f*, 159*f*, 162, 248, 273
Crohn's disease 263
Cryptomenorrhea 184, 185
Cul-de-sac 81, 93*f*, 190, 246, 250, 252
Cystadenocarcinoma
    mucinous 177
    serous 174
Cystadenofibroma 204
Cystadenoma 204
    mucinous 174, 249
    serous 174, 249, 261
Cystic adnexal masses 204
Cystic degeneration 100*f*
Cystic lesions 155
Cystitis 263
    interstitial 233, 235, 238
Cysts 250
    anechoic 155
    complex 161
    endometrial 249
    endometriotic 261
    extraovarian 162*f*
    functional 248, 261, 273
    hemorrhagic 165*f*
    peritoneal inclusion 193
    simple 155

## D

Deep dyspareunia 269
Deep pelvic endometriosis 237
Depression 233, 269
Depth gain compensation 19
Dermatitis 268
Dermoid 172*f*, 173*f*
    cyst 167
Dilation and curettage 288*fc*
Discharge
    causes of 242, 258
    color of 267
    nature of 267
    odour of 267
Diverticular disease 237
Diverticulitis 276
Dominant follicle 87*f*
Doppler effect 21
Double uterus 145*f*, 146*f*
Down syndrome 47
Doxycycline 232
Dysmenorrhea 230, 234, 239, 246,
        254, 264
    evaluation of 242, 266
Dyspareunia 230, 234, 239, 254,
        264, 269
    causes of 242, 268
    clinical evaluation of 242
    superficial 268
Dysuria 235, 239

## E

Ectopic gestations 207
Ectopic implantation
    incidence of 195
    sites of 195
Ectopic pregnancy 46, 136, 185, 195,
        199, 203*f*, 207, 250, 251, 264,
        276, 290*fc*

management of 197
ruptured 208f
sonographic features of 199
Elastography 18
Electronically steered systems 9
Embryo 185
Emergency studies 46
Empty sella syndrome 278
Endocavity ultrasound systems 13
Endocervical growth 259
Endometrial abnormalities 241, 247
Endometrial hyperplasia 121, 221,
  228, 229, 254, 292fc
  clinical evaluation of 242, 272
  history of 242, 272
Endometrial thickness 76f, 117f,
  245, 248, 300
Endometrioid tumor 177
Endometriomas 163f, 204, 264, 273
  bilateral 164f
Endometriosis 230, 233-235, 239,
  240, 269, 277, 297fc
  investigations in 243
Endometritis 120, 120f
Endometrium 57, 76, 77f, 78f, 97,
  100f, 109f-111f, 120, 130f,
  221, 270
  ablation of 228
  atrophic 226, 254
  echogenic irregular 120f
  inflammation of 120
Episiotomy 268
Estrogen deficiency vaginitis 254,
  258
Exercise 278
Extraovarian adnexal areas 58

# F

Fallopian tube 60, 81, 82, 161, 188,
  190, 260
  abnormalities of 185
  carcinoma 189

inflammation of 187
normal 187f
Female pelvis 59
  anatomy of 61f
  normal 69
Fetal
  anomaly 47
  death, misdiagnosis of 46
  heart sounds 212
  parts, absence of 212
Fever 258, 264
Fibroids 97, 119f, 151, 225
  color flow in 97
  complications of 112
  interstitial 106f, 108f
  multiple
    seedling 107f
    submucosal 98f
  number of 97
  pedunculated 204
  polyps 109f
  position of 97
  size of 97
  sonographic evaluation of 295fc
  subserous 106f
  ultrasound features of 104
Fine-needle aspiration cytology 252
Flow direction 24
Flow distortion 28
Flow pattern 25, 27
Flow velocity 25
  waveform 124f
Flow volume 29
Fluid
  collection 117f, 118f, 131f
  debris 250
  endometrial 134
  loculi 58
Foley catheter 151
Follicles 245
  multiple 166
Follicular cyst 160, 248, 273
Follicular monitoring 248

Folliculogenesis 91
Free fluid 58, 250
Frequency 235, 239
  selection 20
Frozen pelvis 277
Full blood count 258
Fundal panmural fibroid 100*f*, 103*f*

## G

Genetic abnormalities 283*fc*
Genital tract
  congenital anomalies of 246
  structural abnormalities of 242, 270
Genital ulcer 254
Germ cell tumors 261, 273
Gestational age 213
Gestational sac 203, 205*f*, 206*f*, 250
  absence of 250
  increased transverse diameter of 213
Gestational trophoblastic neoplasia, development of 214*t*
Gonococcal infection 256, 257
Gram stain 258
Gram-negative diplococci 258
Ground glass appearance 162, 163*f*, 249
Growth 245, 254
  endometrial 259
  retardation 213
Gynecological complications 53
Gynecological diseases, common 241, 282*fc*
Gynecological disorder, history of 239
Gynecological origin, acute abdominal pain of 242, 264
Gynecological pain 289*fc*
Gynecological ultrasound 53
Gynecology
  common symptoms in 241, 253
  Doppler in 54
Gynecomastia 221

## H

Hanafy lens technology 11
Harmonic imaging 16
Heavy menstrual bleeding 234, 270
Hematometra 118*f*, 251
Hematosalpinx 118*f*
Hemoperitoneum 264
  diagnosis of 252
Hemorrhage 162, 250
HIV serology 258
Hormone replacement therapy 222, 229
Hyaline degeneration 99*f*
Hydatidiform mole
  diagnosis of 213*t*
  signs of 212*t*
  symptoms of 212*t*
Hydrocephalus 47, 278
Hydrometrocolpos 116*f*
Hydrosalpinges 233
Hydrosalpinx 189, 191*f*, 204, 251, 260, 277
Hydroureteronephrosis 277
Hyperandrogenism 165
Hyperechoic foci 249
Hyperemesis gravidarum 212
Hyperplasia 253, 270
  benign endometrial 224
Hyperthyroidism 213
  signs of 212
Hypoplastic left heart syndrome 47
Hypoplastic uterus 144*f*
Hypothalamopituitary-ovarian axis 285*f*
Hysterectomy 239
  history of 234
Hysteroscopy 143*f*, 146*f*
Hysterosonogram 223

## I

Incomplete septae 250
Infection 219, 246, 278
Infertility 54, 234, 246, 248, 277
    ultrasound evaluation of 299*fc*
Inflammatory bowel
    disease 233, 236
    syndrome 276
Infundibulum 82
Intermenstrual bleeding 270
Internal iliac vessels 154*f*
Intertrigo 267
Intracardiac transducers 14
Intraluminal transducers 14
Intramural fibroid 98*f*, 107*f*
Intraoperative transducers 14*f*
Intraovarian blood flow 167*f*
Intrauterine adhesions 141*f*
Intrauterine contraceptive device 120, 136, 137*f*, 138*f*, 185, 215, 217, 218
    history of 234
    localization of 246
Intrauterine growth restriction 48
Intrauterine pregnancy 199
    sonographic features of 199
Irritable bowel syndrome 233, 235, 236, 276
Irritable colon 238

## K

Knobology 19, 31

## L

Laminar flow 27
Laparoscopy 164*f*, 198, 240
Left cornual fibroid 104*f*
Left paraovarian cyst 162*f*
Leiomyoma 233, 253, 270
    submucous 248
Leiomyosarcoma 106
Levonorgestrel-containing
    devices 216
Lichen
    planus 267, 268
    sclerosis 268
Limb, absent 47
Loculi, multiple 194*f*
Lost intrauterine contraceptive
    device 218, 220
Low backache 277
Lower abdominal mass 242, 254, 260
    evaluation of 242, 260-262
Low-versus high-resistance flow 26
Lumbar spine, examination of 240
Lymph nodes 245, 252
Lymphadenitis, mesenteric 263
Lymphoma 261

## M

Magnetic resonance imaging 277
Malignancy 253, 270
    diagnosis of 252
Malpractice, causes of 43
Mass 234
    abdominal 240, 252, 254
    complex 250
    descending per vaginum,
        evaluation of 242, 262
    intracavitary 228
    small 245
Medical ultrasound, basic
    principles of 52
Menometrorrhagia 130*f*
Menopausal problems 296*fc*
Menopause 226, 269
Menstrual abnormalities 277
Menstrual cycle 93*f*
    proliferative phase of 85*f*
Menstrual outflow obstruction 278
Menstrual problems 287*fc*

Menstruation after apparent menopause, recurrence of 229
Mesonephric remnants 260
Molar cysts, presence of 211*f*
Molar pregnancy 136
    pelvic ultrasound of 211*f*
Morgagni hydatid cyst 161
Müllerian anomalies, ASRM classification of 241, 244
Müllerian ducts 81
Multicystic ovaries 291*fc*
Multiple cystic spaces 134*f*
Multiple endocervical glands 181*f*
Multiple mature follicles 156*f*
Muscles, spasm of 269
Musculoskeletal disorders 233
Mycobacterium tuberculosis 120
Myofascial pelvic pain syndrome 233
Myoma 247, 251, 260, 272
    anatomical classification of 242, 272
    intracavitary 229
    red degeneration of 264
    submucous 251
Myometrial invasion 248
Myometritis 97, 116
Myometrium 58, 76, 77*f*, 97, 113*f*, 114*f*, 130*f*
    anterior 114*f*
    atrophic 118*f*
    posterior 114*f*

# N

Nabothian cysts 179, 181*f*
Necklace sign 166
Neoplasms, benign 273
Nerve entrapment 233
Neutrophils 258
Noncyclic pain 230
Non-neoplastic ovarian lesions 241, 248

Normal ovary 84*f*, 155*f*, 156*f*, 245
    dimensions of 242, 273
Normal uterus 95*f*
    ultrasonography of 241, 247

# O

Obstruction 115
Obturator internus muscle 154*f*
Oligoovulation 165
Oophorectomy 239
Organs, intra-abdominal 245
Ovarian artery 160*f*
Ovarian cyst 212
    rupture of 264, 276
    torsion of 250, 251, 264, 276
Ovarian dermoid 170*f*, 171*f*, 173*f*
Ovarian disorder 154
    differential diagnosis of 154
Ovarian dysgenesis 278
Ovarian endometrioma 162
Ovarian enlargement, benign conditions causing 242, 273
Ovarian follicle, thick-walled 204
Ovarian follicular cyst, simple 293*fc*
Ovarian fossa 154*f*
Ovarian hyperstimulation syndrome 273
Ovarian malignancy 251
Ovarian mass 241, 252, 277
    evaluation of 178
Ovarian neoplasm 168, 294*fc*
Ovarian pregnancy 207
Ovarian remnant syndrome 233, 236
Ovarian size 300
Ovarian torsion 46
Ovarian tumor 296*fc*
Ovarian volume 91*f*
Ovary 53, 58, 60, 82, 90*f*, 91*f*, 154*f*, 191*f*, 201*f*, 261
    chocolate cyst of 162
    granulosa cell tumor of 254

neoplastic lesions of 241, 249
remnant 234
Ovulation 256
Ovulatory dysfunction 253

## P

Paget's disease 267
Pain
    abdominal 195
    acute 264
    chronic 232
    cyclic exacerbation of 234
    functional 276
    location of 239
    lower abdominal 277
    neuropathic 233
    postoperative 246
    types of 239
Pallor 212
Pancreatitis, acute 263
Panmural fibroid 100*f*, 102*f*
Pap smear 258, 259
Paraovarian cyst 161
Partial hydatidiform mole 213
    diagnosis of 213*t*
Pediculosis 267
Pelvic adhesions 233
Pelvic anatomy, normal 53
Pelvic congestion syndrome 233, 234, 237, 240
Pelvic examination 212, 240, 277
    abnormal 246
Pelvic infection 246
    acute 257
    Doppler studies suggestive of 276
Pelvic inflammatory disease 116, 185, 230, 234, 239, 240, 292*fc*
Pelvic kidney 194*f*
Pelvic mass 240, 247, 252, 254, 277
Pelvic organs, examination of 241, 246
Pelvic pain
    evaluation of 242
    non-gynecological causes of 242, 263
Pelvic sonography 62, 65
Pelvic ultrasonography, techniques for 241, 245
Pelvic viscera 94
    Doppler evaluation of 93
Peptic ulcer, perforated 263
Per rectal examination 240
Per speculum examination 240, 277
Pericystic vascularization 162
Perimetrium 81
Peripheral vessels 103*f*
Peristalsis, active 39
Peritoneal cavity 250
Peritrophoblastic blood flow 206*f*
Pinworm 256
Placenta
    cystic spaces in 213
    previa 47, 49
Polycystic ovary 164, 165, 167*f*, 291*fc*
    syndrome 228, 229
Polyp 132*f*, 133*f*, 152*f*, 229, 245, 247, 251, 253, 254
    abnormality 270
    endometrial 109*f*, 121, 130*f*, 131*f*, 151, 225, 254
    multiple 227
Postcoital bleeding 270
Post-endometrial ablation 229
Posterior wall
    panmural fibroid 99*f*
    submucous fibroid 110*f*, 111*f*
    subserous fibroid 104*f*, 105*f*
Postmenopausal bleeding 245, 248, 270, 298*fc*
    causes of 241, 254
Postmenopausal estrogen deficiency 268

Postmenopausal hormone replacement therapy 227
Postradiation scarring 269
Post-void fullness 235
Pouch of Douglas 58, 93, 190, 192f, 193, 193f, 194f, 197, 245, 269
Power Doppler 33
Pre-eclampsia 212, 213
   signs of 212
Pregnancy 207, 219, 260
   interstitial 205f
   intra-abdominal 207
   test
      negative 221
      positive 264
Previous infection, history of 277
Primary amenorrhea 144f
   causes of 243, 278
   evaluation of 243, 279, 280
Proteinuria 212
Pruritus 254
   vulvae 242, 267
      clinical evaluation of 242, 267
Pseudo sac 197
Psoriasis 267, 268
Psychiatric disorders, history of 239
Psychosomatic disorders 233
Puberty
   delayed 246
   precocious 221, 246
Pubic symphysis, separation of 233
Puborectalis muscle 245
Pulse
   echo 52
      instruments 52
   inversion 16
Pulsed-Doppler transducer 22f
Pus
   aspiration of 252
   drainage of 252
   in cul-de-sac 250
Pyometra 258, 259

Pyoperitoneum, diagnosis of 252
Pyosalpinx 250, 264

## Q

Quality control tests 42

## R

Radiotherapy 279
Range gate cursor 31
Rectovaginal modules 249
Rectovaginal septum 245
Remnant ovary 240
Renal calculus 263
Residual ovary 240
Resistive index 166f
Retroflexion 75
Retroversion 75
Ring of fire pattern 203f
Rokitansky protuberance 167
Rotterdam criteria 164

## S

Sacroiliac joints, examination of 240
Sacroiliitis 233
Saline infusion
   sonography 241, 251
   study 222, 223
Salpingectomy 198
Salpingitis 264
   acute 187
   chronic 188
Salpingostomy 198
Scabies 267
Seborrhea 268
Secondary amenorrhea, evaluation of 243, 281
Sepsis, systemic signs of 264
Sexual dysfunction 233
Shear-wave elastography 19

Simple anechoic functional cyst 157f
Single uterine horn 140
Small intestine 204
Solid ovarian tumor 177
Solid right ovarian mass 177f
Solitary nabothian cyst 182f
Sonohysterography 121, 143, 143f, 150f, 151f
Sound wave propagation 1
Speculum examination 254
Spina bifida, missed 47
STD, history of 234
Stimulation multiple follicles 88f
Stratum
    basale 76
    functionale 76
Stress 278
Stromal tumors 273
Subendometrial flow, moderate 129f
Subendometrial stromal vacuolation 248
Submucosal fibroid 104f, 107f, 110f, 112f
Surgery 268
    history of 239
Swelling 254
Syphilis, serology for 258

## T

Tachycardia 212, 258
Tamoxifen 223, 227
    therapy 248
Tardy reporting 48
Tenderness 231, 254, 264, 277
Teratoma 204
    benign cystic 261
Theca lutein cysts 161, 213, 214, 248, 273
Theoretical training program 51

Thick endometrium 122f-124f, 126f, 127f
Thin endometrium 128f
Thyroid 279
    storm 212
Thyrotoxicosis 212
Tissue
    harmonic imaging 16
    vibration 39
Total hydatidiform mole 210
Transabdominal scan 69, 72f, 172f
Transabdominal sonography 62, 95f
Transabdominal ultrasound 146f, 202f, 208f
Transducer 7
    care 40
    focal zone 6
    formats 15
    frequency 5
    selection 21
Transeophageal echocardiography transducer 13f
Transesophageal transducers 14
Transvaginal scan 69, 145f, 156f, 172f
Transvaginal sonography 62, 73f, 96f, 185, 198
Transvaginal transducer 13f
Transvaginal ultrasound 146f, 206f, 259
Trauma 278
Tremor 212
Trichomonas 268
    vaginalis 256, 257
Trichomoniasis 267
Trilaminar appearance 222
Trophoblastic embolization 212
Tubal evaluation 189
Tubal ligation 235
Tubal surgery, previous 185
Tuberculosis 239, 257
    diagnosis of 252
Tubo-ovarian abscess 167, 250

Tubo-ovarian complex 167, 188
Tubo-ovarian mass 240, 250, 260, 277
Tumors
    endometroid 261
    epithelial 261
    malignant 249
    mucinous 261
Turner syndrome 278
Twin ectopic pregnancies 202*f*

## U

Ultrasonography 162, 213, 241, 248
    basics in 1
    indications for 241, 245
Ultrasound 196
    examination 197
    guided procedures 241, 252
    transducers 12*f*
Ureteric calculus 263
Urethral syndrome 233, 235
Urinary bladder 62
Urinary incontinence 246
Urinary tract infection 276
    chronic 233, 235
    recurrent 235
Uterine 260
    abnormalities 241, 247
    anomalies 247, 248
        congenital 139
    calcifications 116
    cavity 97, 109*f*, 110*f*, 143, 126*f*, 151*f*, 211*f*
    contour 108*f*
        distortion of 104
    corpus 73*f*, 99*f*, 110*f*, 136*f*
    disorders 95
    enlargement 104, 254, 264
    fundus 137*f*
    musculature 97
    myoma, subclassification of 242, 272
    size 300
    synechiae 140
    tenderness 240
    wall, posterior 107
Uterosacral ligaments 240
Uterovaginal agenesis 278
Uterus 53, 57, 59, 69, 72*f*, 79*f*, 80*f*, 96*f*, 117*f*, 201*f*, 213, 246, 250, 278
    acutely retroverted 269
    adenomyotic 113*f*
    anteverted 72*f*-74*f*, 96*f*
    body of 272
    evaluation of 95
    infantile 70*f*
    irregularly enlarged 264
    multiparous 300
    myometrium 106*f*
    nulliparous 300
    postmenopausal 300
    prepuberty 300
    retroverted 74*f*, 75*f*, 269
    septate 122*f*, 146*f*
    size of 97
    subseptate 147*f*

## V

Vagina
    abnormal 183
    lesions of 256
Vaginal atresia 116*f*, 286*f*
Vaginal bleeding 195, 212, 213, 221, 288*fc*
    causes of 225
    irregular 195, 270
Vaginal discharge 240, 242, 253, 254, 259, 267, 269, 276
    causes of 241, 242, 256
    clinical evaluation of 242, 258
    investigations of 242, 257

Vaginal infections, diagnosis of 242, 257
Vaginal swab 240
Vaginal vault 80*f*, 81*f*, 184*f*
Vaginismus 268
    causes of 242, 268
Vaginitis 256, 268
    signs of 269
Venereal disease research laboratory 240
Venous drainage 82, 90
Vesicles, passage of 212
Vesicular mole 260
Vessels, arrangement of 178
Vulva, Paget's disease of 267
Vulval cancer 267
Vulval lesions 268, 269
Vulvar vestibulitis 268
Vulvodynia 268
Vulvovaginitis 256, 267

## W

Wobble sign, positive 169

## X

XX/XY gonadal agenesis 278
XY gonadal agenesis 283*fc*

## Y

Yolk sac 185, 205*f*

EU GSPR Authorised Reprsentative
Logos Europe, 9 rue Nicolas Poussin
1700, La Rochelle, France
Phone: +33 (0) 6 67 93 73 78
E-mail: contact@logoseurope.eu

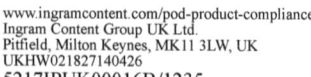